Ultrasound Guidance for Nerve Blocks:

Principles and Practical Implementation

► Except where otherwise stated, drug doses and recommendations are for the non-pregnant adult who is not breast-feeding.

Ultrasound Guidance for Nerve Blocks:

Principles and Practical Implementation

Peter Marhofer

Department of Anaesthesia,
Intensive Care Medicine, and Pain Therapy,
Medical University of Vienna, Austria

With a Foreword by Admir Hadzic

OXFORD
UNIVERSITY PRESS

OXFORD
UNIVERSITY PRESS

Great Clarendon Street, Oxford OX2 6DP

Oxford University Press is a department of the University of Oxford.
It furthers the University's objective of excellence in research, scholarship,
and education by publishing worldwide in

Oxford New York

Auckland Cape Town Dar es Salaam Hong Kong Karachi
Kuala Lumpur Madrid Melbourne Mexico City Nairobi
New Delhi Shanghai Taipei Toronto

With offices in

Argentina Austria Brazil Chile Czech Republic France Greece
Guatemala Hungary Italy Japan Poland Portugal Singapore
South Korea Switzerland Thailand Turkey Ukraine Vietnam

Oxford is a registered trade mark of Oxford University Press
in the UK and in certain other countries

Published in the United States
by Oxford University Press Inc., New York

First published 2008

British Library Cataloguing in Publication Data

Data available

Library of Congress Cataloging in Publication Data

Data available

Typeset by Newgen Imaging Systems (P) Ltd., Chennai, India
Printed in China through Asia Pacific Offset

ISBN 978–0–19–954756–2

10 9 8 7 6 5 4 3

Dedicated to my daughter Melanie

Contributors

Prof. Stephan Kapral, MD
Department of Anaesthesia, Intensive Care Medicine, and Pain Therapy,Medical University of Vienna, Austria

Lukas Kirchmair, MD
Department of Anaesthesia and Intensive Care Medicine, Medical University of Innsbruck, Austria

Manfred Greher, MD
Department of Anaesthesiology, Perioperative Intensive Care, and Pain Therapy, Herz-Jesu Hospital, Vienna, Austria

Prof. Stephan C Kettner, MD
Department of Anaesthesia, Intensive Care Medicine, and Pain Therapy, Medical University of Vienna, Austria

Prof. Harald Willschke, MD
Department of Anaesthesia, Intensive Care Medicine, and Pain Therapy, Medical University of Vienna, Austria

Prof. Christian Czerny, MD
Department of Radiology, Medical University of Vienna, Austria

Mitchell S Kaplan, PhD
Principal Engineer, Advanced Development SonoSite Inc. Bothell, Washington,USA

Contents

Foreword

After decades of lagging behind the improvements made in other anaesthesia subspecialties, regional anaesthesia is undergoing a renaissance. Research efforts prior to the introduction of ultrasound led to improved understanding of functional regional anaesthesia anatomy and regional anaesthesia techniques, the use of nerve stimulators, and longer-acting local anesthetics with safer cardiovascular profiles. However, the single greatest obstacle to the improvement of regional anaesthesia and peripheral nerve block techniques remained the lack of objective monitoring during application of nerve blocks. Modern monitoring allowed general anaesthesia to develop into an exceedingly safe and reproducible medical discipline. In contrast, regional anaesthesia remained a field of a few 'gifted' and superbly skilled enthusiasts. The introduction of ultrasound monitoring during the administration of regional blocks is one of the most significant developments in the history of the subspecialty. With the use of ultrasound, nerve block techniques can be standardized, allowing clinicians to practice with greater degrees of precision and reproducibility. Just as echocardiography is now an essential skill for the cardiovascular anaesthesiologist, ultrasound guidance during the application of peripheral nerve blocks is rapidly becoming a quintessential skill for the modern regional anaesthesiologist.

Ultrasonography provides information that significantly influences the clinical management of the patient. However, acquiring and interpreting this information brings new challenges and responsibilities for the leaders and professional societies in regional anaesthesia. Currently there are limited published data on the advantages of this technology over pre-ultrasound regional anaesthesia techniques. However, based on the already large clinical experience and rapid technological development, it is just a matter of time until the perceived clinical advantages of ultrasound-guided blocks are formally documented in clinical trials. A greater challenge for the future is the development of training criteria and educational standards and the question of a need for certification. In my opinion, the resolution of these challenges is imminent because comprehensive training, including independent work, supervised activities, and assessment programs, is essential for safe and successful practice.

When delving into a new endeavour, the practitioner should always attempt to select the primary source of the information in the topic of interest. Professor Peter Marhofer and his Austrian colleagues are at the forefront of ultrasound-guided regional anaesthesia. For over a decade, they have worked tirelessly to introduce and standardize this technology in regional anaesthesia, making them accomplished teachers and authors on the subject. For these reasons, this volume will undoubtedly play a major role in improving the learning and understanding of ultrasound-guided regional anaesthesia and its wider implementation in clinical practice. It gives me great pleasure to endorse this important publication written by a team of true pioneers with vast clinical and teaching experience. The authors' contributions to more objective monitoring methods during the application of regional anaesthesia is, in my opinion, the only option to promote the more widespread use of regional anaesthesia in the years to come.

Prof. Admir Hadzic,
Consultant Anaesthesiologist,
College of Physicians and Surgeons,
Columbia University,
Director of Regional Anaesthesia,
St. Luke's–Roosevelt Hospital Center

Preface

This book is written by physicians with 15 years' experience in ultrasound-guided regional anaesthesia. Focusing specifically on ultrasound-guided peripheral nerve block techniques, we avoided including basic general knowledge in regional anaesthesia (e.g., indications and contraindications for specific blocks).

We strongly suggest carefully reading the introductory chapters of the book. These include important information about physical background (e.g., to know how to adjust an ultrasound machine in an optimal manner), proven and potential advantages of ultrasound-guided blocks, and prerequisites for practical performance.

The chapters focusing specifically on blocks include precise descriptions about the relevant anatomical considerations (including variations) for each block and practical guidelines for how to perform the blocks in daily clinical practice. Essential information about each block is tabulated at the end of each description (see Table 1 for template).

Illustrations of the typical ultrasound cross-sectional view and the needle guidance technique are provided for each block description. Figures of the needle guidance techniques are shown without a sterile probe cover in order to demonstrate the position of the probe relative to the needle. Where useful, the position of the needle relative to the nerve(s) and/or the distribution of local anaesthetic is also included.

Table 1 Description of specific topics for each particular ultrasound-guided nerve block technique

Block characteristic	Basic, intermediate, or advanced technique (see Appendix 1)
Patient position	Typical position of the patient
Ultrasound equipment	Characteristics of the ultrasound probe
Specific ultrasound setting	Frequency of the ultrasound probe (high – medium – low)
Important anatomical structures	Description of adjacent anatomical structures (vessels, muscles, tendons, etc.)
Ultrasound appearance of neuronal structures	Description of echogenicity and shape of the neuronal structures
Expected Vienna score	Visibility of neuronal structures (see Appendix 2)
Needle equipment	Suggested length and tip of the needle
Technique	Description of the needle orientation relative to the ultrasound probe (in-plane [IP] or out-of-plane [OOP])
Estimated local anaesthetic volume	Suggested volumes of local anaesthetics

Chapter 1

Basic principles of ultrasonography

In order to achieve ultrasound images sufficient for regional anaesthetic peripheral nerve block techniques, some initial considerations about basic principles of ultrasonography are mandatory. The following sections outline essential knowledge about this important topic.

1.1 Nature of sound waves

Sound is the propagation of pressure waves, or an alternating series of localized regions of compression (increased pressure) and rarefaction (decreased pressure) in some material medium (e.g., air or water). Sound waves are *longitudinal*, meaning that the disturbance (alternating compression and rarefaction) occurs along the direction of propagation.

If the propagating disturbance is sinusoidal, the sound wave is composed of a single frequency, f, the rate at which successive compressions or rarefactions occur at a particular location. The units of frequency are the number of compressions (or rarefactions) per second (s), or Hertz (Hz). Besides the propagation direction and frequency, sound waves are characterized by their propagation speed, c, and wavelength, λ. The wavelength of a sound wave is defined as the geometric distance (e.g., in metres, m) between successive regions of compression or rarefaction. Propagation speed depends on the mechanical properties of the medium (density, etc.) and varies considerably across different materials (see Table 1.1). The relationship between propagation speed, frequency, and wavelength is governed by the following equation:

$$c = \lambda f$$

Audible sound (i.e., sound to which the human ear is sensitive) corresponds to frequencies ranging from 20–20,000 Hz. Frequencies above this range are dubbed 'ultrasound', and medical imaging applications typically employ ultrasound frequencies in the range of 1–20 MHz (i.e., up to 1000 times higher than the human ear can hear). Since the speed of sound in human tissue is approximately 1540 m/s, the wavelengths are typically a few tenths of a millimetre.

When sound waves impinge on an interface (a location where the speed of sound changes) or propagate though a dissipative medium, some of the wave energy is scattered or deflected in multiple directions. The original wave is thus attenuated (i.e., loses energy), and the scattered energy ('echoes') carries information about the structure of the medium (e.g., that it contains an interface). It is this information that is ultimately used to create ultrasound images.

Table 1.1 Speed of sound in various materials

Medium	Speed of sound (m/s)
Air	333
Water	1480
Blood	1566
Muscle	1542–1626
Liver	1566
Bone	2070–5350

1.2 Piezoelectric effect

Some materials, notably crystals and certain ceramics, can generate an electrical voltage in response to an applied mechanical stress; these materials also exhibit the converse effect whereby their shape mechanically deforms when subjected to an electrical field. These phenomena are commonly referred to as the *piezoelectric effect*, and this type of material is called piezoelectric material (Figure 1.1).

Figure 1.1 Piezoelectric effect

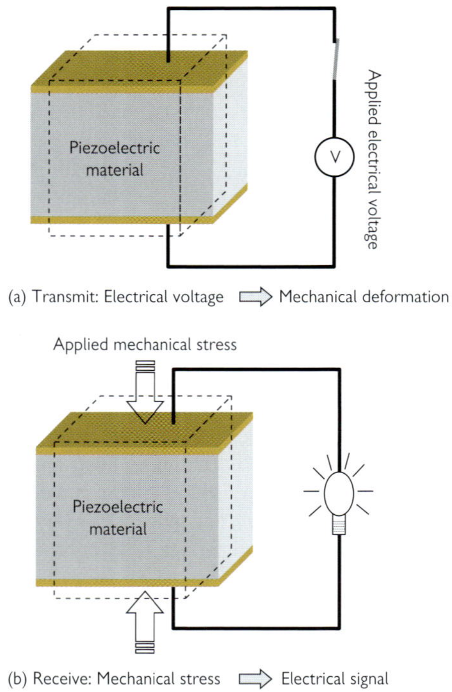

An ultrasonic transducer made out of piezoelectric materials serves as both the sound transmitter and receiver for medical imaging applications. During the sound transmission process, an electric voltage signal (typically up to 100 volts, V, or more) is converted into sound energy (i.e., stress/pressure waves) by the transducer. The generated sound wave then propagates into and interacts with the tissue under examination, and is reflected or scattered by the tissue structure. The energy received from the resulting echoes carries information about the structure, and is converted back into an electrical signal by the transducer for further processing to create ultrasound images that convey the information.

1.3 Pulse-echo instrumentation

Ultrasound images are created by transmitting and receiving a sequence of short pulses along beams spanning an anatomic region of interest (ROI). A typical pulse (relative amplitude versus time) is shown in Figure 1.2. For each pulse, the tissue information at a particular depth is derived from the strength of the received echoes as a function of time. The echoes returned from each transmitted pulse are initially registered as a small voltage (100 mV or less) on the individual piezoelectric elements, which is then amplified and filtered to reduce noise before being digitized with high-precision analogueue-to-digital converters (ADCs). The digital signals from the individual elements are then combined to form a focused *receive beam*. Digital filtering and additional signal processing are employed to calculate the signal power as a function of time, and to produce the image greyscale values along the beam direction.

Figure 1.2 Signal amplitude versus time for a typical pulse used in ultrasound imaging

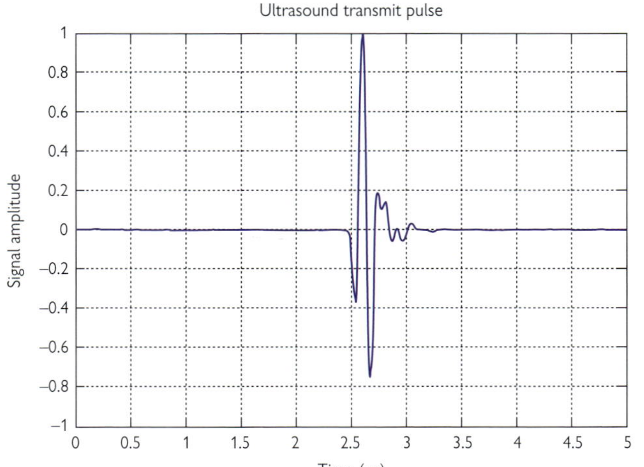

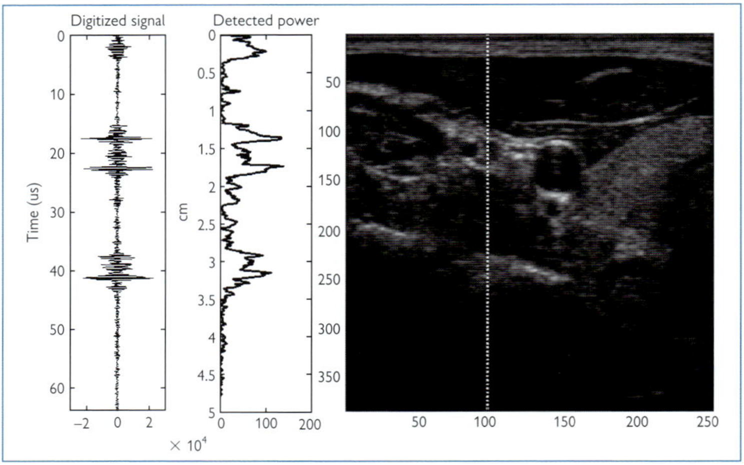

Figure 1.3 Image formation process. The signal from a beam along the dotted line in the image (right) is plotted as a function of time (left), along with the detected power versus the corresponding depth (centre) which is then mapped to a greyscale value in the image. The complete image for a single frame is formed by repeating this process for each beam across the region of interest.

The depth of an echo signal received at a particular time after transmission of the ultrasound pulse can be calculated by assuming an average speed of sound in the body, typically 1540 m/s. For example, a signal received 40 μs after the pulse transmission corresponds to a depth of 3.08 cm (20 μs travel time each way × 1540 m/s = 0.0308 m = 3.08 cm).

The image formation process is depicted in Figure 1.3, where the signal from a beam along the dotted line in the image on the right is plotted as a function of time (left), along with the detected power versus the corresponding depth (centre). The detected power values are then mapped to image greyscale values versus depth. This is repeated for each beam across the ROI to complete the image for a single frame.

1.4 Resolution and electronic focusing

The utility of medical images is largely determined by how well various features may be identified and distinguished from each other and from the background. The *resolution* of an image quantifies the minimum distance required between two features for them to be discriminated, and may be expressed in terms of several individual components, including axial, lateral, contrast, and temporal resolution.

Axial resolution (i.e., along the line of acoustic propagation) is primarily determined by the length of the transmitted pulse. Figure 1.4 illustrates what happens when the distance between two features approaches the pulse length:

Figure 1.4 Envelope of received signal from axially-resolved (left) and unresolved (right) pins

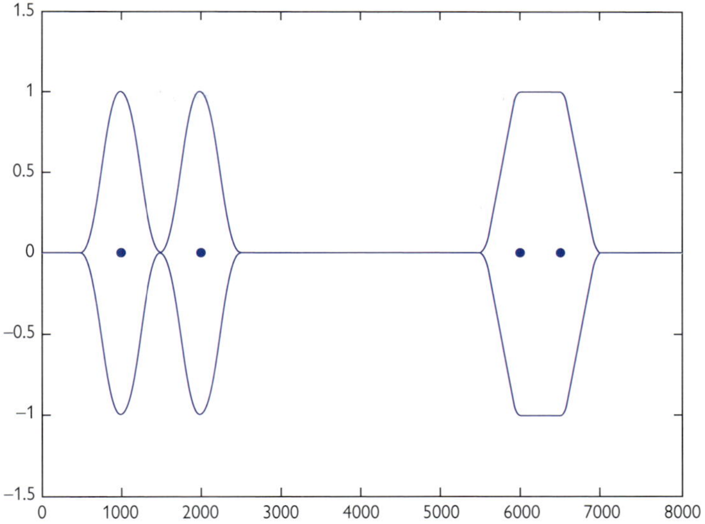

they appear to fuse into a single, thicker feature, and are therefore not resolved. Higher-frequency transducers generally provide better axial resolution because higher frequencies imply shorter wavelengths, which allow shorter pulse lengths. Longer pulses are sometimes employed to increase penetration or sensitivity (since they have more energy) at the cost of degraded axial resolution.

Lateral resolution (i.e., perpendicular to the direction of acoustic propagation) is primarily determined by the focusing power of the transmit and receive beams. Typical two-dimensional (2D) ultrasound transducers consist of an array of individual elements arranged along a common plane, wherein each element transmits and receives ultrasound energy over a wide range of angles. To construct an image, the data from the elements are combined to form beams that focus the energy to a very narrow range of angles. This is accomplished for both transmit and receive beams by summing delayed versions of the signals from the various elements. As illustrated in Figure 1.5, the delays are designed so that the propagation times from all elements to the focal point are identical. Transmit beams are focused at one of a few (typically 1–4) focal depths in the image; each requires a separate pulse, so frame rate is sacrificed for the improved resolution provided by additional transmit focal zones. Upon reception, the delays are adjusted 'dynamically' so that every point along the beam is a receive focal point.

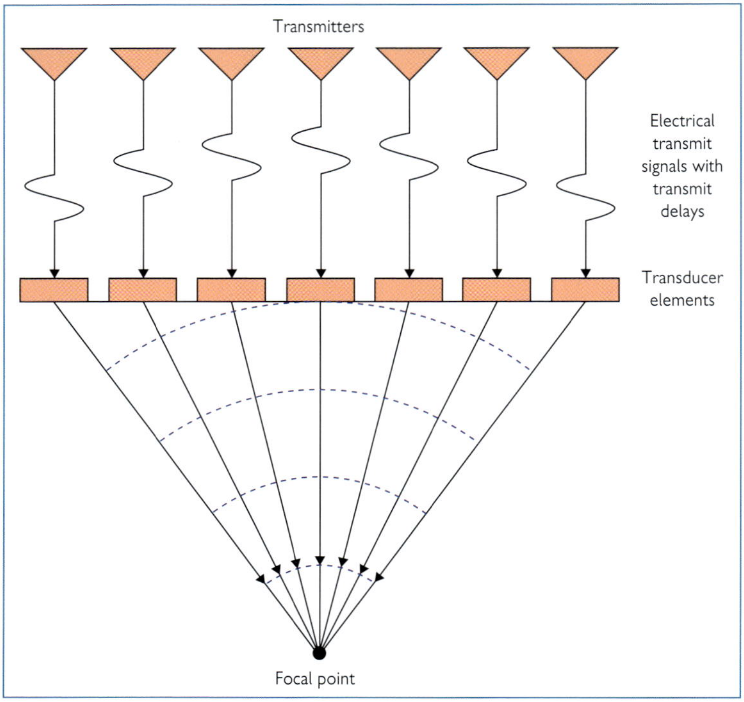

Figure 1.5 To focus an ultrasound beam on transmission, the outer elements are pulsed before the inner elements, so that the sound pulses from each element arrive at the focal point at the same time. When receiving, the signals from outer elements are delayed relative to the inner elements before summing to compensate for the longer ultrasound path length.

Contrast resolution is the ability to distinguish regions of different acoustic reflectivity, as observed in the intensity or greyscale presentation of the image.

Temporal resolution is the ability to track motion from frame to frame, and is primarily determined by the frame rate.

1.5 Time-gain compensation

As an ultrasound pulse propagates through tissue, some of its energy is scattered and absorbed, reducing the energy of the pulse as well as of the echoes used to form an image. Because this attenuation causes the received signal to decrease with increasing depth, an amplifier with time-dependent gain is typically used to compensate, ensuring that the analogue signal amplitude remains in a reasonable range and preventing a reduction in image intensity with depth. As illustrated in Table 1.2, attenuation varies considerably across

Table 1.2 Ultrasound attenuation in various tissues	
Tissues	**Attenuation (dB/cm/MHz)**
Water	0.0002
Blood	0.18
Soft tissues	0.3–0.8
Brain	0.3–0.5
Liver	0.4–0.7
Fat	0.5–1.8
Muscle	0.2–0.6
Tendon	0.9–1.1
Bone	13–26
Lung	40

different tissue types, and is usually quantified in terms of decibels (dB) per cm per MHz (where the frequency refers to the average frequency of the pulse). Typically, an average attenuation of approximately 0.5 dB/cm/MHz is assumed to establish the default time-gain compensation (TGC), which can be as much as 60 dB (1000-fold amplification) or more. Because attenuation varies so much with anatomy, etc., user-adjustable controls are common. Slide controls, for example, may allow the user to modify the gain at different depths to 'even out' the image intensity. Alternatively, some systems provide an automatic gain feature that analyses the image data and automatically adjusts the gain as a function of depth, as shown in Figure 1.6.

1.6 Measuring velocity with pulsed ultrasound

The velocity of an ultrasound scatterer (e.g., a blood particle) moving along the ultrasound beam direction may be measured by correlating the reflected pulse echoes from successive transmissions ('pings'). In practice, this is accomplished by sequentially transmitting a number of beams along a fixed direction with a carefully selected, constant time interval between them. The time interval (*pulse repetition interval*, or PRI), or equivalently its inverse, the *pulse repetition frequency* (PRF), determines the velocity range that can be unambiguously estimated. For a given ultrasound frequency, the velocity range increases with increasing PRF. Ultimately, the PRF (and therefore the maximum measurable velocity) is limited by the round-trip acoustic travel time to the depth of interest because a second pulse cannot be transmitted until the first has been fully received.

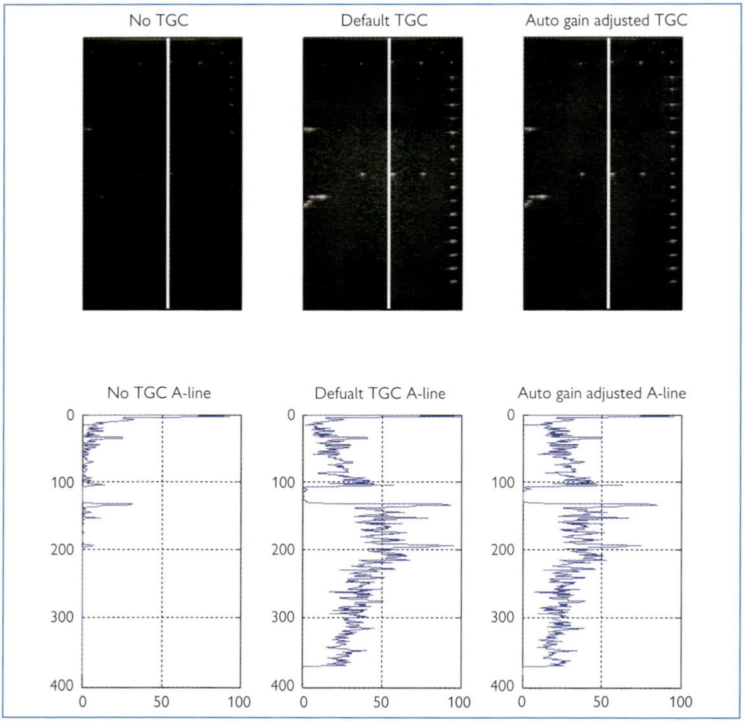

Figure 1.6 Phantom images (top) and profiles (bottom) showing the effects of attenuation with no time-gain compensation (left), default time-gain compensation (centre), and time-gain compensation after automatic adjustment (right)

Figure 1.7 illustrates how the pulse correlation technique works for two example cases: a scatterer moving away from the transducer with a relatively high velocity (top panel) and a relatively low velocity (bottom panel). For each, a series of received echoes is displayed (left panel). Successive pulses are shifted in time relative to their predecessors because the object from which they are reflected is moving away from the transducer. The time shift is greater for the fast-moving scatterer because it moves farther during the interval between successive pings. The right panel shows the pulse amplitude at a particular point, relative to the transmission time. These amplitude samples trace out a sinusoidal pattern with respect to the pulse index, and the frequency of the sinusoid is directly proportional to the velocity of the scatterer. Ultrasound systems employ sophisticated signal processing methods to extract this information from a sequence of pulses and use it to compute and display the spatial distribution of average velocity (*colour-flow* or *colour-velocity imaging*) or the velocity distribution of a collection of scatterers at a particular spatial location as a function of time (*spectral Doppler imaging*).

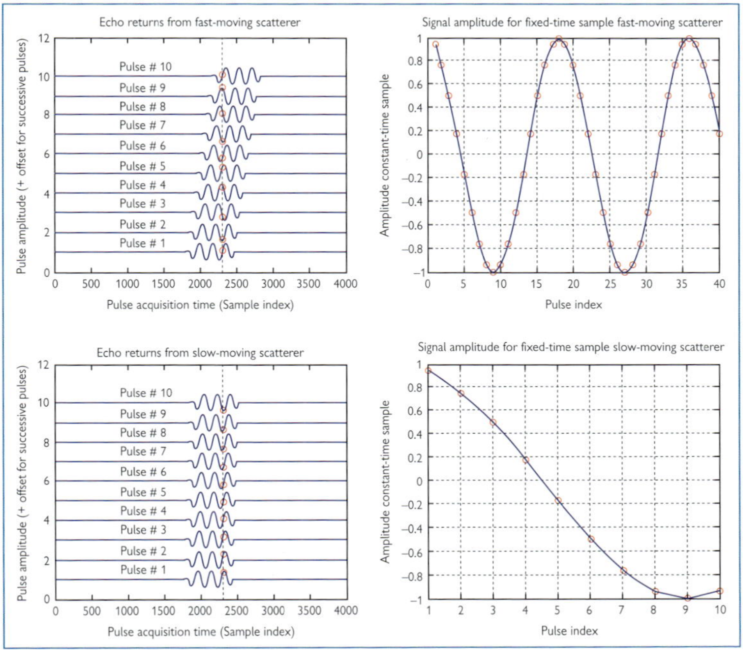

Figure 1.7 Left: Received echo (RF) time series reflected from a particle moving away from the transducer with relatively high velocity (top) and relatively low velocity (bottom). Right: Pulse amplitude at a fixed time relative to the transmission time for the pulses shown on the left. The frequency of the resulting sinusoid is proportional to the particle velocity.

1.7 Ultrasound imaging modes

Modern scanners present ultrasound data to doctors and sonographers in various forms. The most common is the sonogram, or *B-mode* image. An example is shown in Figure 1.8, where the 2D sector image is similar to a black and white picture of an anatomical slice.

M mode is a specialized case of B-mode imaging where one particular line (the 'm-line') is ensonified repeatedly, with the resulting greyscale information displayed as a scrolling image so that the same location is seen as it changes in time. An example is shown in Figure 1.9.

In *C mode*, the (directional) blood velocity is estimated within a ROI and encoded as a colour image superimposed on the B-mode greyscale image, as shown in Figure 1.10. An alternative to this colour-velocity imaging is colour-flow imaging, in which the power of the blood-flow signal may be displayed instead of the velocity.

Figure 1.8 B-mode image of liver and kidney

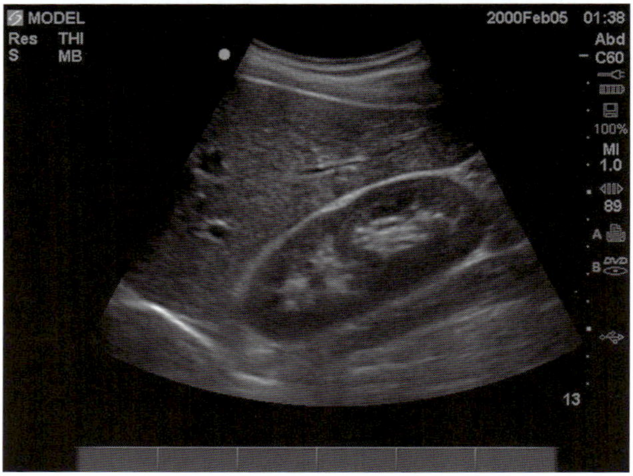

Figure 1.9 M-mode image of a foetal heart

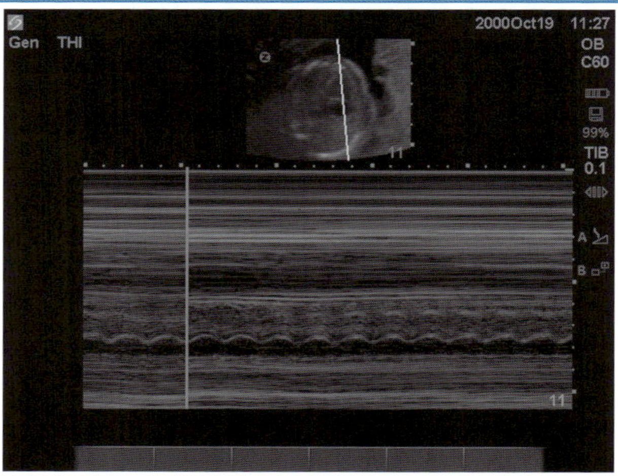

An example of a *D mode*, or spectral Doppler, image is shown in Figure 1.11. The lower portion of the figure shows a scrolling greyscale image depicting the velocity distribution of the blood at a particular location (the *sample volume*) versus time. The vertical axis of the scrolling data represents blood velocity and the intensity (greyscale) indicates the strength of the blood flow-signal. Pulsed-wave (PW) Doppler velocity ranges are limited by the depth of the sample volume.

Figure 1.10 Umbilical cord showing blood flow. Red and blue imply blood flow away from and towards the transducer, respectively

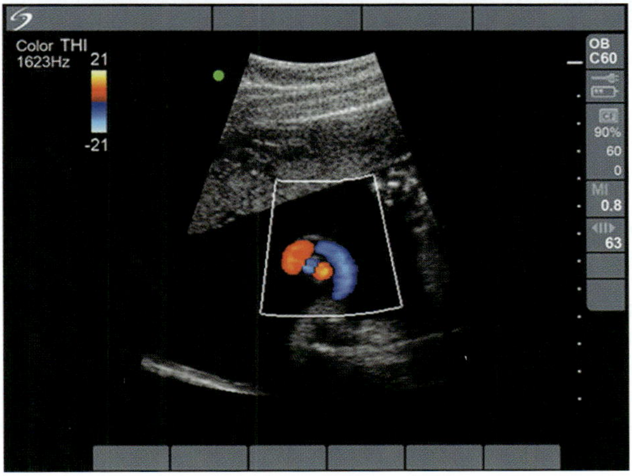

Figure 1.11 Arterial flow in the carotid measured with spectral Doppler

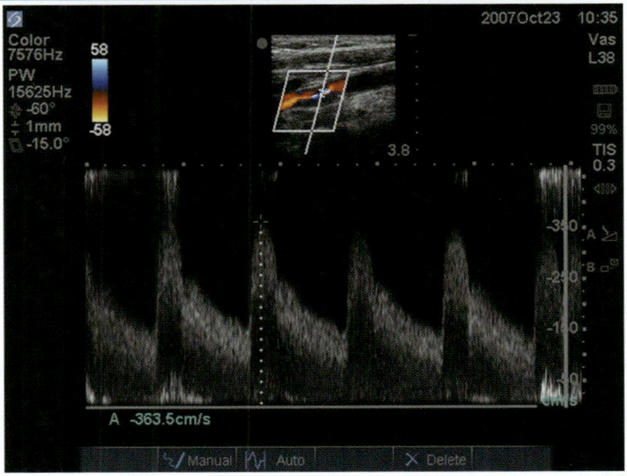

In continuous-wave (CW) Doppler imaging, no sample volume is selected. Indeed, it is not possible to specify a time/range gate, so the velocity distribution displayed is sensitive to all depths along the selected direction. CW mode is used when the velocity range required is not accessible with PW, as often occurs in cardiac applications. A CW Doppler image is displayed using the same format as a PW Doppler image.

Other modalities that are increasingly common include 3D (which takes several contiguous B-mode slices and stacks them together to create a volume image), contrast imaging, and elastography.

1.8 Common Image Artefacts

There are a number of common image artefacts that often degrade ultrasound image quality, including speckle, clutter, reverberation, and aliasing (for colour-flow and spectral Doppler).

Speckle is a very characteristic texture commonly seen in ultrasound images. It is essentially an interference pattern superimposed on the 'true' image arising from scatterers that are too small and closely spaced to be resolved. Because the pattern depends on angle, it can be suppressed by combining images acquired with multiple steered ultrasound beams (spatial compounding), as shown in Figure 1.12.

Although the focusing techniques discussed above result in beams with very narrow main lobes, there may still be significant sensitivity to ultrasound energy arriving from particular directions outside of the main beam (e.g., from side or grating lobes). Echoes received from these directions will be misplaced in the image and contribute to clutter artefacts, particularly in hypoechoic regions such as vessels, amniotic fluid, cysts, and bladders. Tissue harmonic imaging (THI) and aperture apodization are frequently used to reduce these artefacts. Figure 1.13 shows how THI reduces clutter in the gall bladder.

Reverberation is produced when a strong ultrasound signal is reflected back and forth between two or more interfaces with large acoustic impedance differences, such as at a tissue–gas or tissue–fluid interface. The artifact typically appears as a repeated pattern of an anatomic feature. As shown in Figure 1.14, re-orienting the ultrasound beam (rotating or tilting the transducer) and/or reducing the gain may reduce reverberation artefacts.

Velocity aliasing is the most common artifact seen in colour-flow and spectral Doppler images. When the actual flow velocity is faster than a PRF can support, the aliased velocity wraps around and shows up at the opposite end of the frequency axis, as shown in Figure 1.15. A similar effect in colour-velocity images appears as artefactual reversed directional flow. Aliasing can be avoided by increasing the PRF.

Figure 1.12 Much of the speckle in a conventional ultrasound image (left) is suppressed in the corresponding image acquired with spatial compounding (right)

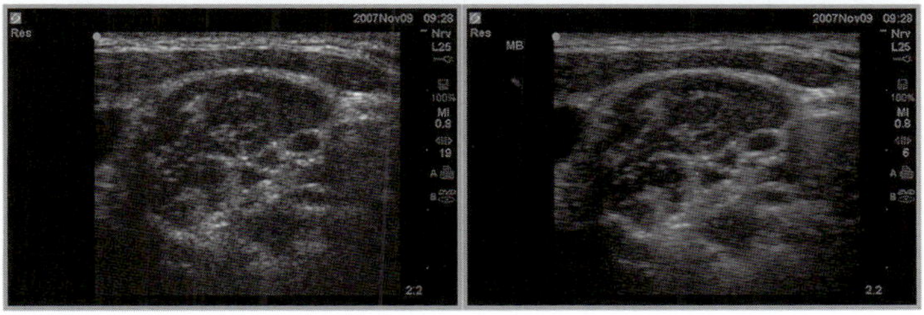

Figure 1.13 The clutter (low-level greys) visible in the gall bladder (left) is significantly reduced in the image acquired with tissue harmonic imaging (right)

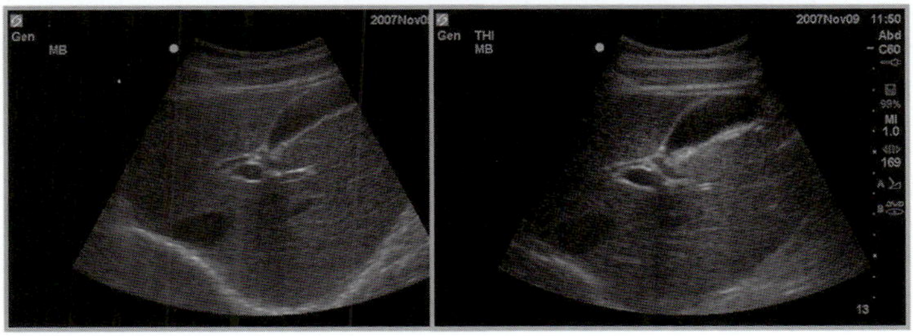

Figure 1.14 The strong reverberation artefact that appears inside the vessel (left) may be reduced either by decreasing the gain (centre) or by tilting the transducer (right)

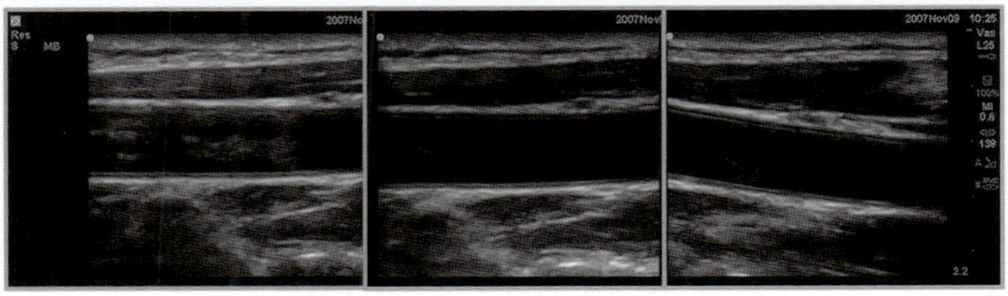

Figure 1.15 By increasing colour-velocity and Doppler pulse repetition frequency to proper scales, the velocity aliasing artefact (left) is diminished (right) in both imaging modes

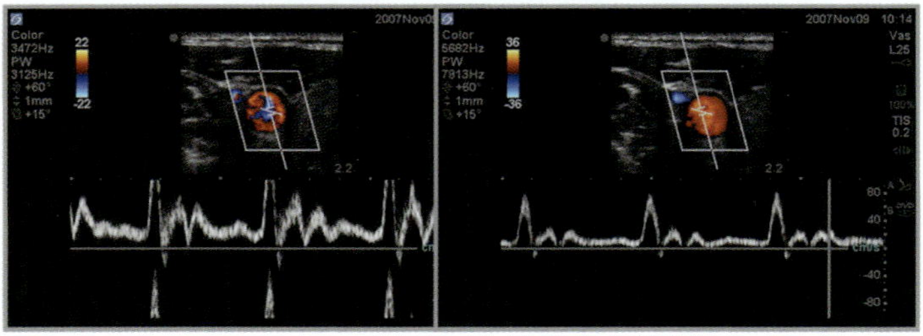

1.9 Equipment needed for ultrasound imaging

Three pieces of equipment are needed for ultrasound imaging: (1) an imaging system; (2) a transducer (also known as a 'scanhead' or 'probe'); and (3) transmission gel. The system itself consists of a front-end subsystem that orchestrates the transmission signalling and reception of the reflected echoes. Transmission signalling includes pulse characteristics (e.g., centre frequency, length, amplitude), transmit beam-forming, and the order in which beams are transmitted to compose an imaging frame. Reception includes TGC, analogue filtering, receive beam-forming, analogue-to-digital conversion, digital filtering, and various amounts of mode-specific signal processing. Additional processing is typically required to condition the data for display. System software is also required: (1) to provide a user interface that allows the user to select imaging mode, depth, exam type, etc.; (2) to configure the various system components based on these inputs; (3) to provide connectivity (e.g., internet, USB, etc.); and (4) to perform various calculations based on the ultrasound data and/or additional user inputs.

Three types of transducers are used for the vast majority of 2D ultrasound imaging applications: (1) linear arrays (Figure 1.16); (2) curved arrays (Figure 1.17); and (3) phased arrays. High-frequency probes provide superior spatial resolution, whereas low-frequency probes offer greater penetration. Linear arrays are typically used to produce images with a finely-sampled, rectangular field of view, whereas curved arrays are typically used to produce a diverging 'sector-shaped' field-of-view that expands beyond the lateral extent of the transducer. Phased arrays often provide a linear array 'form factor' with the expanding field of view that is characteristic of curved arrays.

Figure 1.16 25- and 38-mm linear ultrasound probes (both 6–13 MHz)

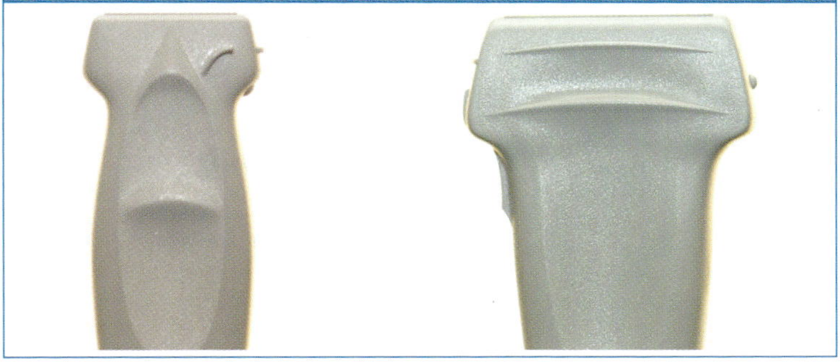

Figure 1.17 Curved array probe (2–5 MHz)

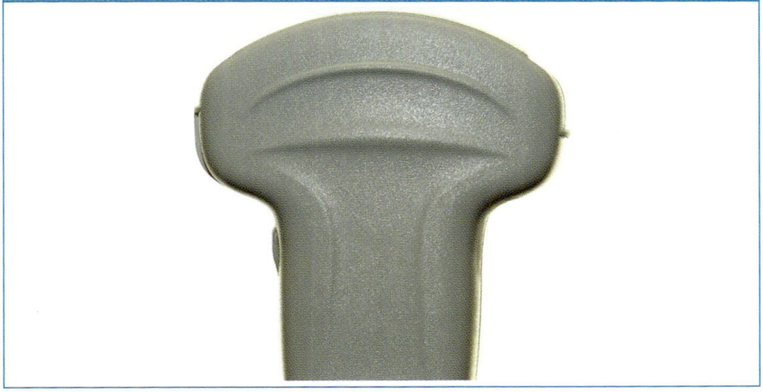

Transmission gel is essential for ultrasound imaging. Without it, there would inevitably be an air gap between the surface of the transducer and the patient. Because the speed of sound is so different in air, most of the ultrasound energy would be reflected from this interface and would not propagate into the patient. Gel provides a coupling medium that efficiently transmits ultrasound energy from the transducer to the patient and vice versa.

Further reading

Sites B, Brull R, Chan V *et al.* Artifacts and pitfall errors associated with ultrasound-guided regional anaesthesia. Part 1: Understanding the basic principles of ultrasound physics and machine operations. *Regional Anesthesia and Pain Medicine* 2007; **32**: 412–418.

Chapter 2

Initial thoughts and potential advantages of regional anaesthesia under ultrasonographic guidance

Since 1884, when Carl Koller described the first successful blockade of a peripheral nerve in Vienna, regional anaesthesia has become an important specialty for providing adequate perioperative pain control. Nevertheless, a close evaluation of significant advantages during the past decades is disappointing. The introduction of the most recent new local anaesthetic drug was roughly a decade ago, and the same situation could be presumed for additive substances.

A similar situation can be observed for guidance techniques. All reported techniques until the early 1990s are based on indirect methods, such as pure landmark-based techniques, nerve stimulation, or surface mapping. These methods postulate either that morphometric measurements are applicable on a large population or that the position of tip of the needle is an indicator for a successful blockade. Both assumptions have never been confirmed by validated scientific methods. Indeed, scientific publications show that anatomy is highly individual – a logical explanation for the poor success rates of some peripheral regional anaesthetic techniques. Another reason for such disappointing success rates might be that the tip of the needle might block the nerve structures. It sounds simple, but the distribution of local anaesthetic is after all the main factor for successful blockade.

In 1994, Kapral *et al.* published the first paper investigating the use of direct ultrasonographic visualization during a peripheral plexus block technique (*Anesth Analg* 1994). Even with suboptimal ultrasound equipment at that time it was possible to directly evaluate the correct distribution of local anaesthetic around nerve structures of the supraclavicular brachial plexus. This was the beginning of a new area in regional anaesthesia: direct visualization. Since then, ultrasound equipment has improved dramatically and, in parallel with this, so has our knowledge and skills in terms of nerve visualization. Today, probe frequencies of 13 MHz or more are available even for transportable ultrasound equipment, allowing us to visualize tiny nerves and other anatomical structures.

The main argument against ultrasound guidance for regional techniques is the lack of large randomized studies comparing complications of ultrasound guidance with other techniques. As the complication rate of regional anaesthesia is nowadays very low, such studies would have to include thousands of patients.

Thus, we have to accept that these large outcome studies will not be available in the near future, if they are to be realized at all. We should therefore try to find an acceptable midpoint between 'evidence-based' and 'expert-based' medicine concerning the use of ultrasound-guided regional anaesthesia.

The overall number of scientific studies in the field of ultrasonography in regional anaesthesia has increased dramatically. However, it is very difficult to distinguish between poor- and high-quality studies. Over the course of scientific evaluation of this technique, many different methods and opinions have been published. An intensive dialogue between the proponents has led to the unification of most of the techniques, such that only anatomically meaningful techniques should now be used in daily clinical practice. Several advantages of ultrasound-guided regional blocks have been described in a number of well designed studies and confirmed in clinical practice. These include:

Safe identification of neuronal structures

With the ultrasound equipment now available, identification of even the smallest neuronal structures is possible. Nevertheless, adequate technique remains an important prerequisite, with individual knowledge and hand skills of equal importance. A high level of experience with ultrasonography is the most important factor for the safe identification of neuronal structures. Every nerve has a particular visualization in ultrasonography, and the form and echogenicity of this may vary at different anatomical ROIs.

Identification of adjacent anatomical structures

Of particular importance for establishing safe and effective nerve blocks is to identify any relevant adjacent anatomical structures such as vessels, bones, tendons, muscles, or pleura. Therefore, good anatomical knowledge and the ability for 3D imagination are mandatory to avoid complications and to predetermine the spread of local anaesthetic.

Observation of the spread of local anaesthetic

It is often forgotten that it is the local anaesthetic solution which blocks the nerve, and that the distribution of local anaesthetic cannot be reliably predicted with indirect needle guidance techniques. Indeed, direct observation of the spread of local anaesthetic is one of the main advantages of ultrasonography. In cases of maldistribution of local anaesthetic, needle replacement is always possible in order to achieve adequate spread.

Observation of the needle

In addition to ensuring adequate spread of local anaesthetic, direct observation of the needle is an important factor in avoiding complications. Whether the entire needle can be visualized in its entirety or only at the tip depends on the block technique being used (IP versus OOP). Both techniques have their specific indications with associated advantages and problems (see Chapter 6). Although it is frequently stated in this book that the local anaesthetic and not the tip of the needle provides a successful nerve block, direct visualization of the tip of the needle is mandatory for a successful block and to safely avoid complications (e.g., nerve puncture or damage of adjacent anatomical structures). This requirement is independent of whether an IP or OOP technique is used.

Faster onset times and longer duration of blocks

Because of the close administration of local anaesthetic to nerve structures, the onset times of ultrasound-guided blocks are significantly shorter compared with conventional techniques. It has also been shown that the duration of blocks is significantly longer following ultrasound-guided techniques. These improvements in block characteristics are based on exact administration of local anaesthetic, and are mainly independent of the volume of local anaesthetic that is used.

Painless performance of blocks

Ideally, regional anaesthesia is performed in a painless manner. With the sole exception of ultrasound guidance, all current techniques are based on physical interaction with nerves (e.g., paraesthesia techniques, nerve stimulation) and are therefore associated with uncomfortable sensations. Furthermore, muscle response during nerve stimulation is a painful procedure in cases of traumas (e.g., luxation of joints, fractures). In addition, the smaller volumes of local anaesthetic required for ultrasound-guided techniques compared with conventional methods, along with the subsequent reduction in pressure forces, may provide superior comfort for patients during blockade.

Reduced volumes of local anaesthetics

In addition to its pain-sparing benefits, reducing the volume of local anaesthetic used in nerve blockade also increases the safety of the procedure. Several studies have shown that blocks using 20–30% of previously recommended local anaesthetic volumes are possible under direct visualization of the nerve structures. It seems that large volumes have been used in the past to compensate for inexact guidance techniques. Reviewing the literature, one can still find recommendations to administer 40 mL of local anaesthetic for interscalene or axillary brachial plexus blocks. As a consequence, side effects such as co-blockade of the phrenic nerve may occur during interscalene blockade. In addition, low (or adequate) administration of local anaesthetics reduces the risk of systemic toxicity; patients with impaired cardiovascular function may profit from low plasma levels of local anaesthetics. This is also true in children, in whom low levels of binding proteins can cause increased toxicity of local anaesthetics.

Low complication rates and high success rates with reduced conversions to alternative anaesthetic methods

Give these potential advantages of ultrasound-guided regional anaesthesia should result in low rates of complications and high rates of success. However, as mentioned earlier, it is extremely difficult to provide adequately rigorous scientific evidence for the observed reduction of complication rates with ultrasound-guided methods in comparison with conventional techniques. Our knowledge about nerve physiology is still not sufficient to understand all the mechanisms of nerve damage and potential dangers of electrostimulation or direct nerve puncture. Nevertheless, it seems to be an appropriate concept to avoid needle–nerve contact in order to prevent nerve damage. In any case, direct visualization of all anatomical structures involved in the blockade increases the safety of regional techniques, avoiding damage to these structures during puncture. Despite a lack of adequate clinical trials, this concept for avoiding complications appears convincing.

By review of the literature, an overall success rate of 80% for peripheral regional techniques with conventional guidance techniques is described. This implicates a large number of block failures and subsequently high conversion rates to alternative methods. Conversion to general anaesthesia is associated with patient discomfort and increased incidence of complications. In addition, the necessity of a second anaesthesia method is uneconomical.

Further reading

Eichenberger U, Stöckli S, Marhofer P, Huber G, Willimann P, Kettner SC, Pleiner J, Curatolo M, Kapral S. Dose reduction of local anesthesia for peripheral nerve blocks: a newer ultrasound-guided, nerve diameter based method. *Regional Anesthesia and Pain Medicine (at press).*

Hopkins P. Ultrasound as a gold standard in regional anaesthesia. *British Journal of Anaesthesia* 2007; **98**: 299–301.

Horlocker T and Wedel T. Ultrasound-guided regional anesthesia: in search of the holy grail. *Anesthesia and Analgesia* 2007; **104**: 1009–1011.

Kapral S, Krafft P, Eibenberger K, Fitzgerald R, Gosch M, Weinstabl C. Ultrasound-guided supraclavicular approach for regional anaesthesia of the brachial plexus. *Anesthesia and Analgesia* 1994; **78**: 507–513.

Marhofer P and Chan V. Ultrasound-guided regional anesthesia: current concepts and future trends. *Anesthesia and Analgesia* 2007; **104**: 1265–1269.

Chapter 3

Limitations of the technique

Every serious analysis of a new method should also consider its potential limitations. For ultrasound-guided regional anaesthesia, these can be divided into technical and non-technical limitations.

3.1 Technical limitations

Physical law dictates that the deeper the anatomical structures, the lower the ultrasound frequencies needed to visualize them. Therefore, direct nerve visualization for deep blocks, such as psoas compartment blockade, is not always possible. Nevertheless, the identification of adjacent structures (e.g., the lower pole of the kidney during psoas compartment blockade) increases the margin of safety for deep blocks.

Not all regional techniques are meaningful under ultrasound guidance. A questionable regional technique for ultrasound guidance is epidural anaesthesia in adults. Since most of the neuraxial structures are surrounded and protected by bones, the ultrasound visualization of the epidural space is extremely difficult and, in some cases, almost impossible. Despite extensive scientific and practical efforts of experienced users, ultrasound guidance for placement of epidural catheters has not found its way into daily clinical practice. Whereas in children all neuraxial structures are clearly visible (Figure 3.1), albeit in an age- and weight-dependent manner, ultrasonography of neuraxial structures in adults is disappointing and, in most cases, of minor clinical importance (Figure 3.2).

3.2 Non-technical limitations

In addition to these technical limitations of ultrasound-guided regional anaesthesia, one of the main challenges to increasing its usage in clinical practice is that anaesthesiologists have to change their mind. It is difficult to convince those who have worked for several years with alternative methods of nerve identification during regional blocks. Indeed, it is easy to find arguments against new techniques and several years of intensive scientific and practical evaluation are usually needed to introduce a new technique in widespread clinical practice.

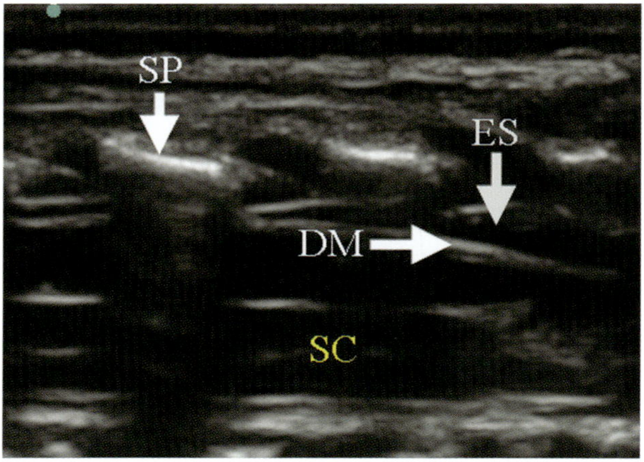

Figure 3.1 Ultrasonographic appearance of the neuraxial structures in a 3-kg baby (left side = cranial). DM: dura mater; ES; epidural space, pictured caudally and filled with local anaesthetic; SC: spinal cord; SP: spinous process).

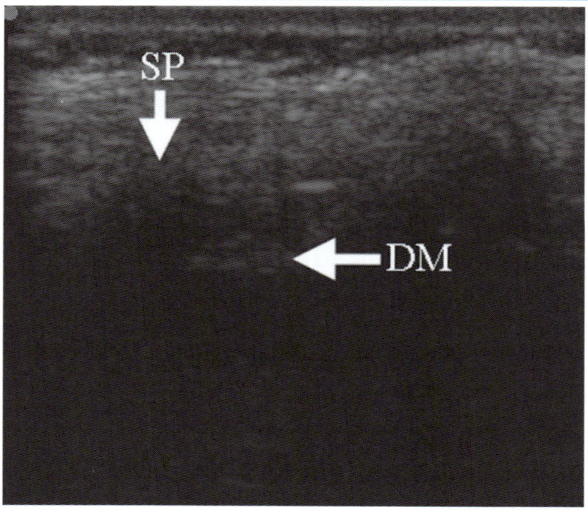

Figure 3.2 Ultrasonographic appearance of the dural mater (DM) at the lumbar level in an adult (left side = cranial). SP: spinous process.

A prerequisite for adequate use of a new technique is intensive education. In recent years, several useful workshops have been established all over the world, both as part of anaesthesia congresses and as independent, highly specialized workshops (e.g., www.sono-nerve.com, www.nysora.com, etc.). However, the optimal method by which to introduce ultrasound-guided regional blockade to daily clinical practice remains under discussion. It is rather difficult to provide close supervision by experienced users for the high number of potential and interested anaesthesiologists and institutions. Therefore, optimal learning tools are prerequisites and an absolute necessity for novices and those with limited experience. Useful learning tools include DVDs that demonstrate practical block techniques, and books, which should be published by experienced users.

Nevertheless, close supervision for those who intend to start with this technique should be part of an educational framework. In recent years, the number of practical users has constantly grown, resulting in great improvements across the field. In addition, guidelines for the adequate use of ultrasound-guided regional anaesthesia and recommendations on how to start are now available; these should serve as a basic introduction to the technique.

Further reading

Grau T, Leipold R, Delorme S, Martin E, and Motsch J. Ultrasound imaging of the thoracic epidural space. *Regional Anesthesia and Pain Medicine* 2002; **27**: 200–206.

Willschke H, Bösenberg A, Marhofer P *et al.* Epidural catheter placement in neonates: sonoanatomy and feasibility of ultrasonographic guidance in term and preterm neonates. *Regional Anesthesia and Pain Medicine* 2007; **32**: 34–40.

Chapter 4

Technical and organizational prerequisites for ultrasound-guided nerve blocks

Some important issues should be considered prior to the introduction of ultrasound-guided regional anaesthesia in daily clinical practice. It is of particular importance to highlight the necessity of considering technical and organizational requirements for the adequate and optimal use of this technique and its initial introduction.

4.1 Technical considerations

4.1.1 Optimal equipment

Every institution and individual physician should carefully decide which ultrasound equipment is optimal for their purposes. Since the advent of portable equipment, ultrasound machines have become much more affordable and, due to intensive research, the image quality of portable machines is now similar to larger and more expensive ones. Nevertheless, the initial costs for ultrasound equipment are significant, even for relatively low-priced machines. It is therefore necessary to calculate the overall costs for this new and innovative technique, taking into consideration aspects of an individual institution.

Due to enormous interest in ultrasound-guided regional anaesthesia, some manufacturers have designed specialized equipment adapted specifically for the purposes of visualization of nerves. We have found that it is cost effective to avoid nonspecific software and/or tools and to focus on one specific indication. In cases when a machine is shared with other subspecialties (e.g., intensive care), additional software might be useful. All in all, additional costs should not be an insurmountable problem in providing optimal care for our patients.

4.1.2 Needle equipment

The appropriate ultrasonographic visibility of needles is an important consideration. Nevertheless, enhancement of needle visualization in ultrasonography has been overstated. Although several manufacturers have designed needles specifically for ultrasound purposes by using different materials or surfaces, no needle has yet been shown to have a particular advantage over other needles. In fact, the better the visibility of a needle, the more image artefacts are caused.

More importantly, we should consider the following factors of needle visibility:

- *Diameter of the needle*: The larger the needle size, the better the visibility, but the more image artefacts are caused.
- *The angle of insertion*: A flat angle of insertion provides better visualization when an IP technique is used, whereas a steep angle of insertion causes impaired needle visualization.
- *Tip of the needle*: It has been shown that needles with facette tips allow optimal movement in tissues. The facette tip is relatively sharp (Figure 4.1), and therefore exact placement is facilitated in comparison with blunt needles (e.g., Sprotte needles).
- *Injection line*: In order to realize an 'immobile needle technique' according to Winnie (*Anesthesiology*, 1969) an injection line is mandatory (Figure 4.2). A technique where the syringe is directly connected to the needle is associated with inadvertent needle movement and is therefore inexact.

In summary, there is currently no evidence for significant advantages of so-called 'ultrasound needles'. Nevertheless, we use ultrasound products in our daily clinical practice because we have found them to be cost effective. The avoidance of an electric cable for nerve stimulation purposes and an isolated shaft may significantly lower the costs once these needles are produced in large numbers.

Figure 4.1 22-G needle with a Facette tip

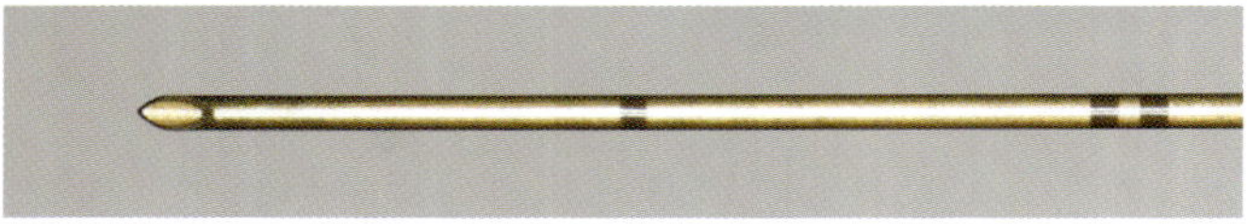

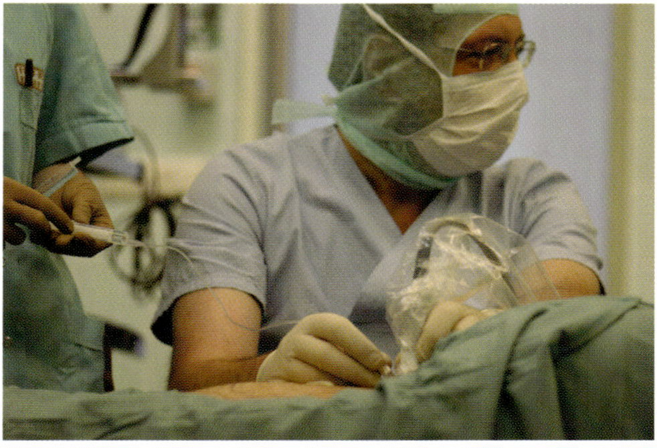

Figure 4.2 Immobile needle technique according to Winnie where the practitioner holds the ultrasound probe in one hand and moves the needle with the other hand and a second person administers the local anaesthetic solution following the instructions of the practitioner.

4.1.3 **Sterility**

Sterile preparation of the probe and the block area is a prerequisite for ultrasound-guided block techniques. Subspecialties such as interventional radiology have been using covered probes for many years in order to preserve sterility. Despite their extensive experience with ultrasound-guided interventions, an optimal cover has yet to be identified.

The expert statement paper, published in 2007 (see Appendix 1 for a summary), recommends a sterile probe cover for single and continuous block techniques. Figure 4.3 shows the latest development in that field, where a transparent adhesive sheet is connected to a plastic foil. This unique arrangement of two different materials avoids getting jelly between the probe and the cover. Of course, (sterile) jelly between the probe cover and the skin is necessary. We have found that urinary catheter jelly can be used as an alternative to dedicated and more expensive sterile ultrasound products, and that the use of only one jelly layer improves the picture quality significantly.

Figures 4.4–4.7 illustrate how the sterile ultrasound probe cover should be used.

Figure 4.3 Sterile probe cover system with a transparent adhesive sheet (below) connected to a plastic foil

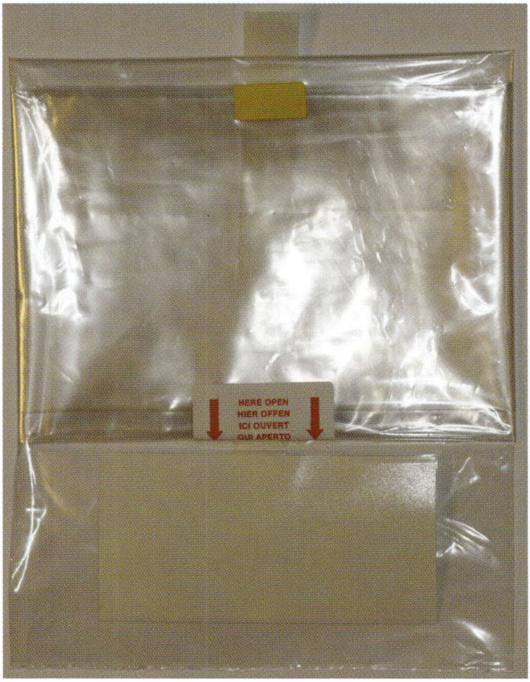

Figure 4.4 Correct use of the sterile probe cover. The 38-mm active area of the linear probe is placed on the adhesive part of the probe cover

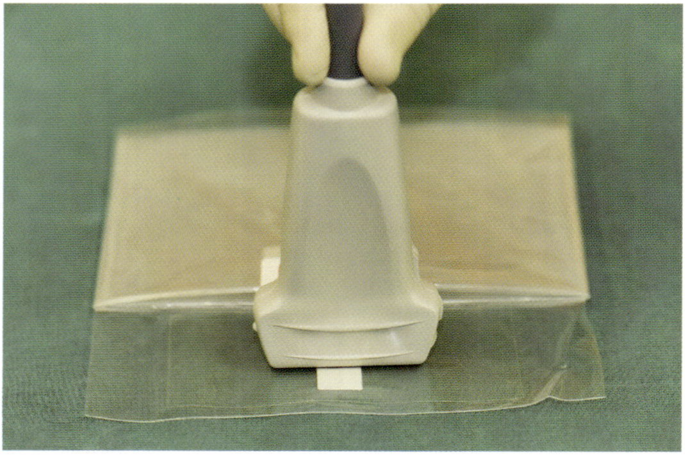

Figure 4.5 Correct use of the sterile probe cover. The probe is covered all over by the plastic sheath

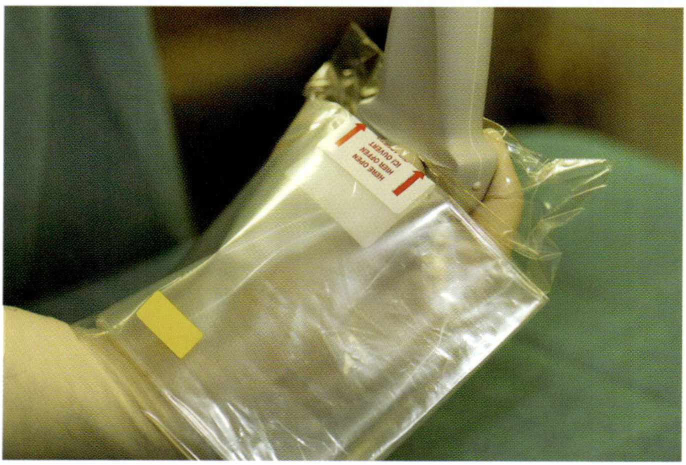

Figure 4.6 The ultrasound probe and the cable is covered in a sterile manner

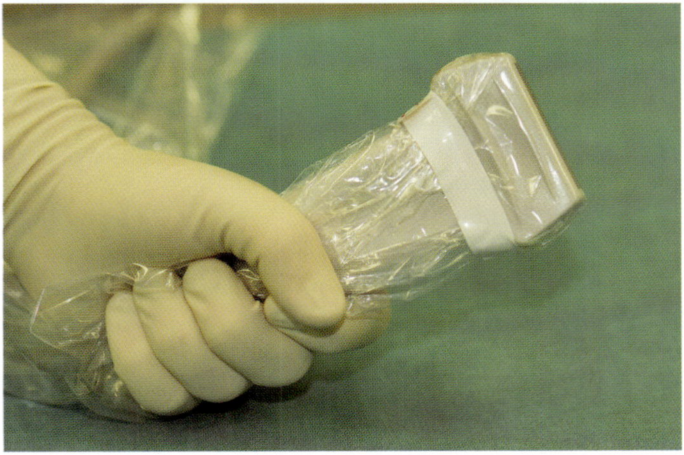

Figure 4.7 The active area of the ultrasound probe with the sterile probe cover. It is important and easily possible to avoid any creases in order to maintain optimal image quality

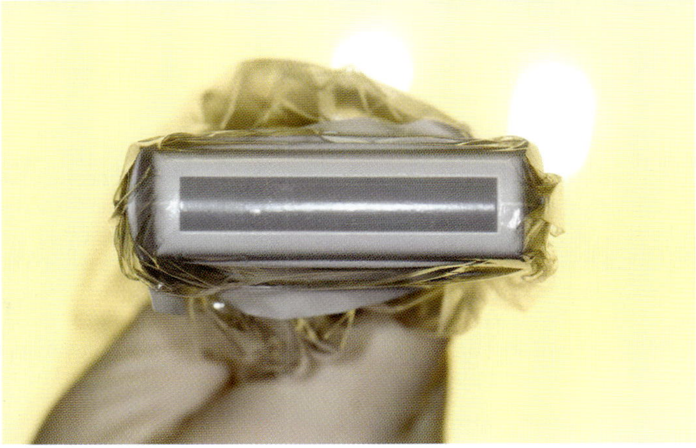

4.2 Organizational considerations

4.2.1 How to start?

There is still no worldwide consensus about optimal training for beginners interested in ultrasound-guided regional blocks, nor for the introduction of these techniques in their daily clinical practice. It is far beyond the scope of this book to discuss all aspects of training, education, learning tools, and eventual certification. Instead we provide a simple but reliable statement to facilitate getting started with the technology.

Theoretical prerequisites

- Basic knowledge of ultrasound physics and machine adjustment.
- Basic anatomy and sonoantomy of the relevant areas of interest.

Once the necessary theoretical knowledge has been acquired, a basic workshop should be visited. Nearly all anaesthesia congresses provide these basic workshops, where experienced specialists demonstrate scanning techniques. The next step should be the acquirement of practical abilities.

Practical prerequisites

- Understanding of needle guidance techniques.
- Beginners should master level 1 blocks (see Appendix 1 for definition) before attempting more complex techniques.

Once basic block techniques can be performed in a safe and successful manner, an advanced workshop should be visited. These workshops should provide intensive hands-on training in combination with teaching 'deeper' theoretical knowledge (e.g., anatomical variations). Continuous training is necessary for optimizing one's own hand skills. The learning curves are highly individual, but we have found in our daily clinical practice that level 2 block techniques are able to be managed by most anaesthesiologists.

4.2.2 Where should we perform the block?

Whether regional nerve blocks are performed in or out of the operating room (OR) depends on the internal organization of institutions. In our experience with both locations, we have found that the advantage of a dedicated 'block room' is that it can be adapted to suit the specific purposes of regional blocks. After nerve blockade, the patient can be transported into the OR and the surgical procedure can start without delay, resulting in a smooth OR process. Giving proper consideration to the onset and duration of blockade allows for more efficient time management.

4.2.3 Postoperative observation

Optimal patient care also includes post-anaesthesia care. In our experience over the past decade, we have observed that ultrasound-guided block techniques reduces the length of stay in the post-anaesthesia care unit. Due to the improved block qualities in comparison with conventional techniques, as well as extremely low conversion rates to general anaesthetic techniques, most patients can bypass the post-anaesthesia care unit altogether. Patients can be transferred straight to the ward or even directly to their home, which is cost effective and improves patient comfort.

4.3 Other considerations

4.3.1 Monitoring

Minimal demands for monitoring during the performance of ultrasound-guided blocks are:

- Intravenous line.
- Pulse oximetry.
- Electrocardiogram.
- Blood pressure monitoring.

Dependent on the medical status of the patient and the surgical procedure additional monitoring might be necessary.

Further reading

Maecken T, Zenz M, and Grau T. Ultrasound characteristics of needles for regional Anesthesia. *Regional Anaesthesia and Pain Medicine* 2007; **32**: 440–447.

Chapter 5

Ultrasonographic appearance of nerves and other anatomical structures

Adequate interpretation of all anatomical structures in ultrasonography is a prerequisite for the correct performance of regional techniques.

5.1 Appearance of nerves in ultrasonography

Recall that 'every nerve has a particular visualiztion in ultrasonography'. This statement may sound confusing, but it reflects our observations during the past decade.

On analyzing a histological illustration of a peripheral nerve, the epineurium, perineurium, connective tissues, and neurons are visible. By using high-frequency ultrasonography the visualization of all those structures is possible (Figure 5.1).

Figure 5.1 Histological and corresponding ultrasound illustration of a peripheral nerve

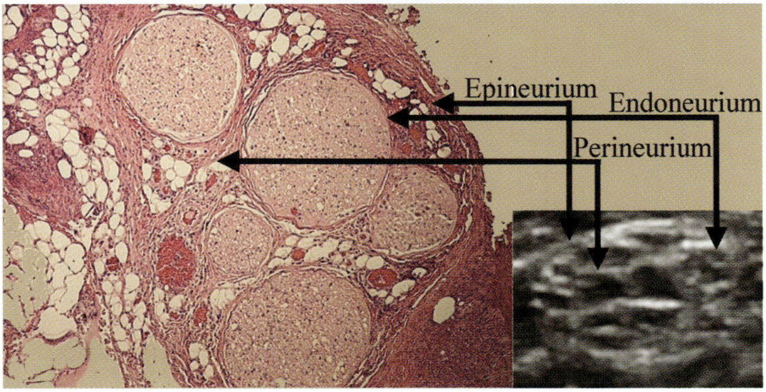

Due to a large percentage of neuronal structures, when visualized in a proximal position nerve structures appear hypoechoic with a hyperechoic surrounding (Figure 5.2). The more peripheral the visualized nerve structures, the more hyperechoic the image (Figure 5.3), which can be explained by the increased percentage of connective tissue between neurons.

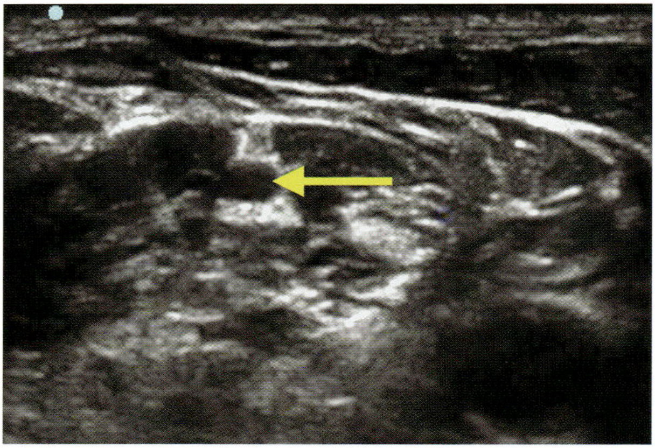

Figure 5.2 The arrow indicates a hypoechoic central nerve structure (C5 root in the interscalene space) with a hyperechoic border in the area of the interscalene groove. Tracking this nerve structure in a proximal and distal direction is possible and is an important method of identification.

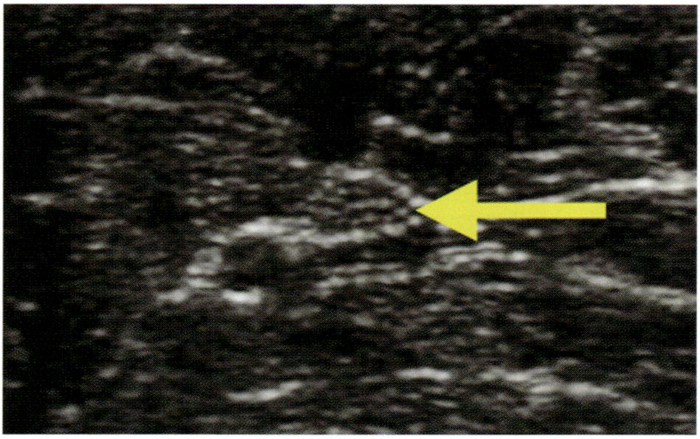

Figure 5.3 The arrow indicates a hyperechoic peripheral nerve structure (ulnar nerve at the level of the lower third of the forearm). Tracking this nerve structure in a proximal and distal direction is possible and an important method of identification.

For the purposes of regional anaesthesia, nerves should always be visualized in a transversal view, appearing as described above. In principle, it is also possible to visualize nerves in a longitudinal view, wherein the internal echotexture is described as a reticular pattern in which longitudinal discontinuous bands are visible (Figure 5.4). In daily clinical practice, however, the longitudinal view is of minor importance.

It is an interesting phenomenon that nerves appear in different forms depending on their anatomical position. One example is the ulnar nerve in the distal upper arm position, at the proximal and the middle forearm (Figure 5.5). Some nerves have a constant typical form, including the musculocutaneus and radial nerves, but, in principle, all peripheral nerves appear in individual and typical forms. These forms can be described as round (Figure 5.6), oval (Figure 5.7), or triangular (Figure 5.8). The correct description of the ultrasound appearance of peripheral nerves is therefore based on both echogenicity and form (e.g., hyperechoic and round).

Figure 5.4 Longitudinal view of a peripheral nerve

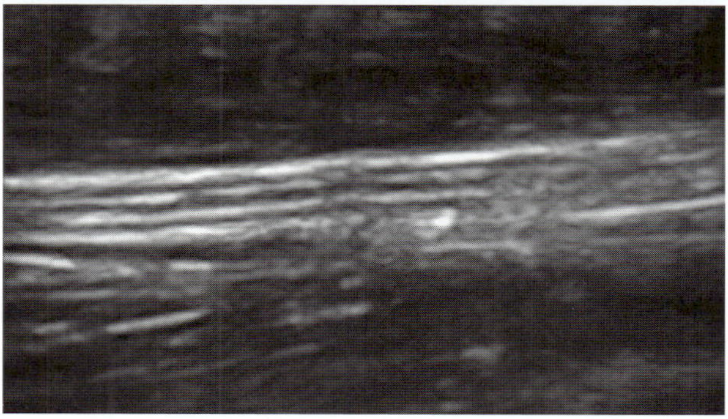

Figure 5.5 Typical form of ulnar nerve at three different anatomical positions (above the elbow joint → oval; proximal third of the forearm → triangular; distal third of the forearm → round)

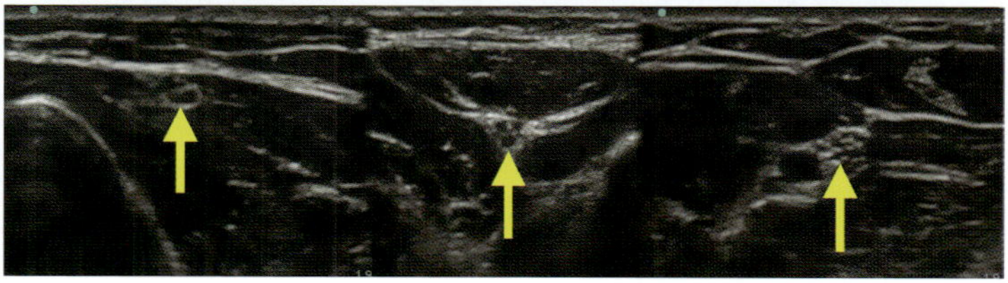

The angle of the probe relative to the nerves is also important. The echogenicity of structures varies according to the angle of the ultrasound beam, a phenomenon known as *anisotropy*. The anisotropic behaviour of peripheral nerves is individual, with the sciatic nerve showing the highest level of variation (Figure 5.9).

For certain regional anaesthetic techniques, nerve structures are not directly visible under ultrasound guidance. In these cases, distinct anatomical knowledge is a prerequisite for successful performance of the blockade (e.g., rectus sheath of intercostal nerve blocks).

Figure 5.6 Round shape of a peripheral nerve (tibial nerve at the popliteal level)

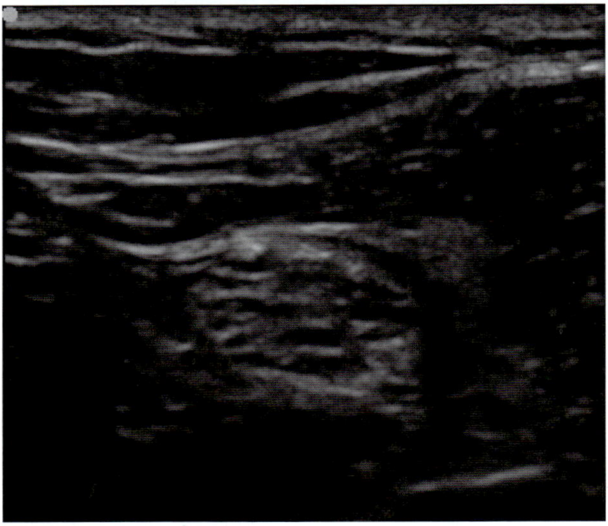

Figure 5.7 Oval shape of a peripheral nerve (sciatic nerve at the midfemoral level)

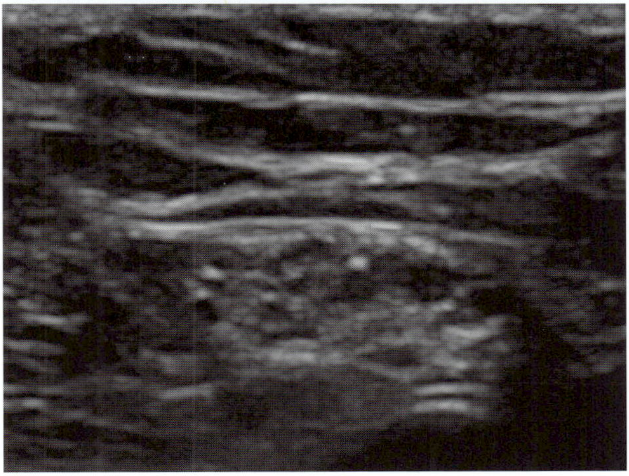

Figure 5.8 Triangular shape of a peripheral nerve (ulnar nerve at the level of the forearm)

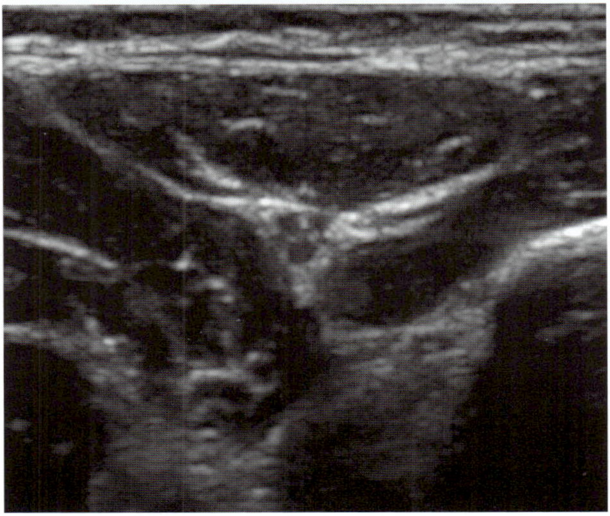

Figure 5.9 Anisotropic behaviour of a peripheral nerve. Left: the sciatic nerve is clearly visible; Right: the sciatic nerve disappears after a 5° movement of the ultrasound probe

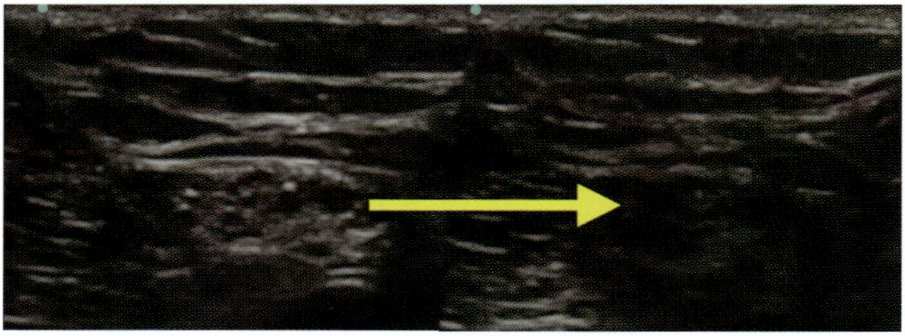

5.2 Appearance of other anatomical structures in ultrasonography

In addition to correct ultrasound-guided interpretation of peripheral neuronal structures, it is also important to correctly recognize adjacent anatomical structures. This particular knowledge is mandatory for correct performance of blocks and to avoid complications.

5.2.1 Tendons

In a transverse view the ultrasonographic appearance of tendons is similar to those of nerves (Figure 5.10). An excellent method for clear discrimination of these structures is to track them over a certain distance: whereas tendons disappear over distances, nerves should be visible in their entirety. Using a longitudinal view, the internal structure of tendons is visualized as longitudinal continuous hypoechoic bands with hyperechoic intertendinous septae (Figure 5.11, fibrillar pattern).

5.2.2 Blood vessels

The safe identification of blood vessels is of particular importance. Discrimination of arteries and veins is possible with colour Doppler imaging (Figure 5.12). An additional and simple method to discriminate arteries from veins is to increase the contact pressure of the probe: veins are compressible but arteries retain their rounded shape (Figure 5.13). However, a practical implication of this is that there is a risk of inadvertent and unnoticed puncture of the vein due to high probe-related contact pressure. Direct observation of the spread of local anaesthetic during injection is absolutely mandatory to avoid intravascular drug administration.

Figure 5.10 Cross-sectional view of a nerve (yellow arrow) and a tendon (white arrow). Discrimination is only possible by tracking the structures in a proximal direction, whereupon the tendon disappears

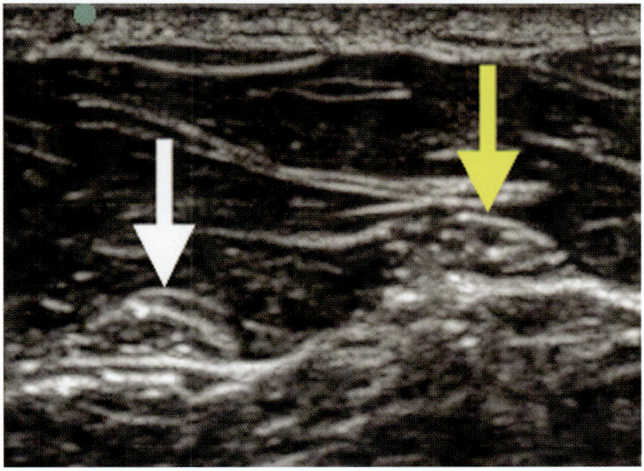

Figure 5.11 Typical longitudinal view of a tendon

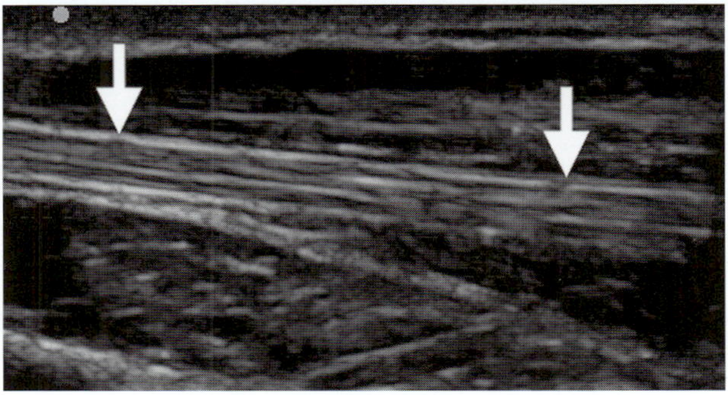

Figure 5.12 Colour Doppler of the femoral vein (right side = blue) and artery (left side = red)

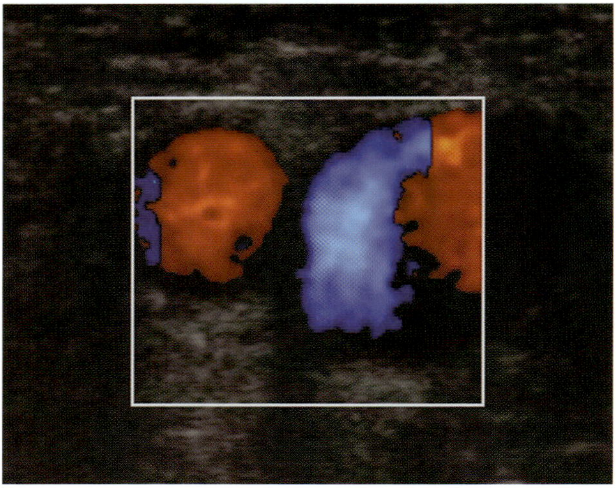

Figure 5.13 Non compressed (left side) and compressed (right side) femoral vessels (red arrow = artery; blue arrow = vein)

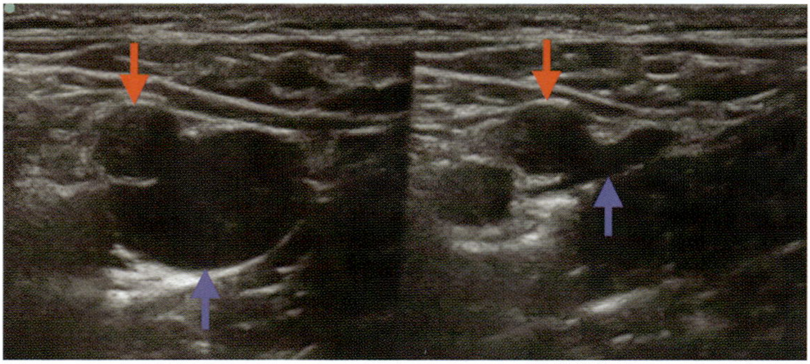

Blood vessels can also serve as guidance structures to facilitate the location of nerves. The infraclavicular portion of the brachial plexus or the femoral nerve lateral the femoral artery are prime examples.

5.2.3 Muscles

Muscles may appear in ultrasound images either as slightly heterogeneous structures with band-like hyperechoic intramuscular septae (Figure 5.14) or as homogeneous structures (Figure 5.15). In general, muscles show a fibrolameller ultrasonographic appearance. Muscle tissue is often the main reference structure regarding echogenicity of nerves. It is helpful to assign the different muscle structures relative to the nerves.

Figure 5.14 Heterogeneous muscle appearance with band-like hyperechoic intramuscular septae

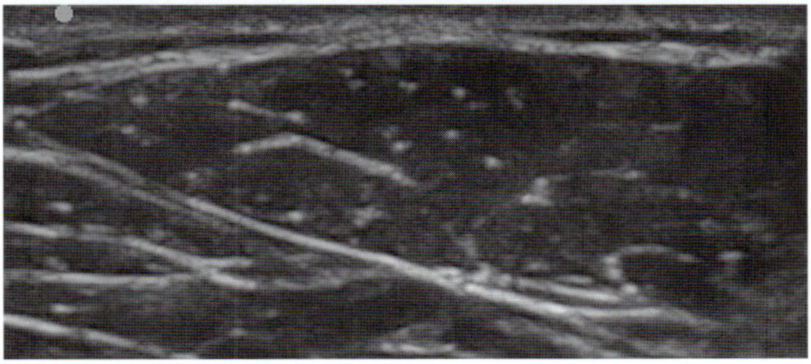

Figure 5.15 Homogeneous muscle appearance

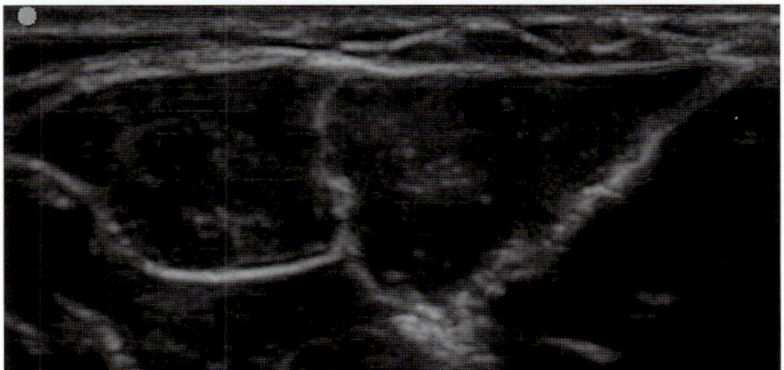

5.2.4 Bones

In general, bony structures cannot be evaluated with ultrasonography. The cortex appears as a hyperechoic structure, and the contour of cortex may serve as a guidance structure for specific block techniques (e.g., deep cervical plexus blockade). Due to the fact that the ultrasound beam is totally reflected by the cortex, the areas behind the cortex are completely anechoic (dorsal ultrasound shadow). Figure 5.16 illustrates the appearance of a bony structure in ultrasonography.

5.2.5 Lymph nodes

Lymph nodes appear oval- or bean-shaped with a hyperechoic vascularized hilus entering the lymph node from its border. Lymph nodes are typically depicted as having a longitudinal diameter of 2–3 mm. Reactive lymph nodes are usually slightly enlarged with delineating hilus structures, and of oval appearance. Malignant lymph nodes are usually round, show no hilus structures, and have a low echogenicity.

5.2.6 Local anaesthetic

Local anaesthetic solution appears anechoic in ultrasonography (Figure 5.17). Improved identification of nerve structures is often possible after administration of local anaesthetic.

5.2.7 Air

Air bubbles appear as hyperechoic artefacts with dorsal shadows (Figure 5.18). Co-administration of air bubbles during blocks should therefore always be avoided due to impaired visualization of anatomical structures.

Figure 5.16 Ultrasonographic appearance of the humerus, where the cortex of the bone appears hyperechoic with an anechoic dorsal ultrasound shadow

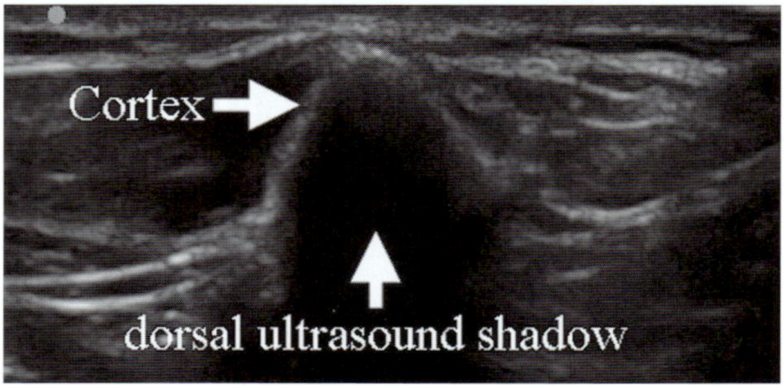

Figure 5.17 Ultrasonographic visualization of local anaesthetic (yellow arrow = nerve; white arrow = hypoechoic appearance of local anaesthetic)

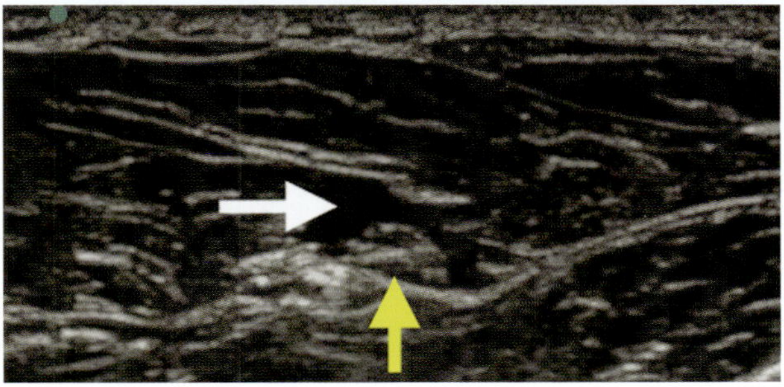

Figure 5.18 Ultrasonographic appearance of air bubbles (white arrow) with dorsal shadow

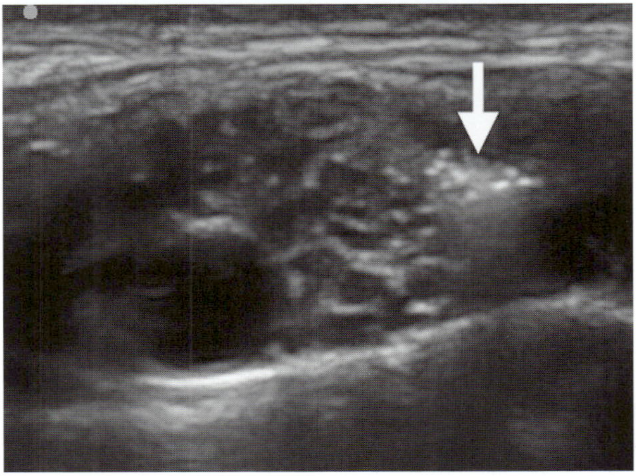

Further reading

Sites B, Brull R, Chan V *et al.* Artifacts and pitfall errors associated with ultrasound-guided Regional Anaesthesia. Part II: A pictorial approach to understanding and avoidance. *Regional Anesthesia and Pain Medicine* 2007; **32**: 419–433.

Chapter 6

Needle guidance techniques

As we have seen, there are two different needle guidance techniques used for ultrasound-guided nerve blocks: out-of-plane (OOP) and in-plane (IP). These techniques describe the position of the needle relative to the ultrasound probe. In principle, both techniques can be used for most blocks, but anatomical implications require that each specific block technique should be preferentially performed with IP or OOP.

6.1 Out-of-plane needle guidance

In the OOP technique, the needle is positioned along the short axis of the ultrasound probe (Figure 6.1). Depending on the depth of the target structure, the angle of the needle has to be adjusted. A flat angle is suitable for superficial target structures, whereas deep target structures require steeper angles. Only the tip of the needle can be visualized by using the OOP technique (Figure 6.2). Nevertheless, the OOP technique is preferred for most of the blocks we will encounter later (e.g., interscalene approach, infraclavicular approach, peripheral blocks of the upper extremity, femoral nerve block, ilioinguinal/iliohypogastric nerve blocks, etc.).

Figure 6.1 Out-of-plane position of the needle relative to the ultrasound probe

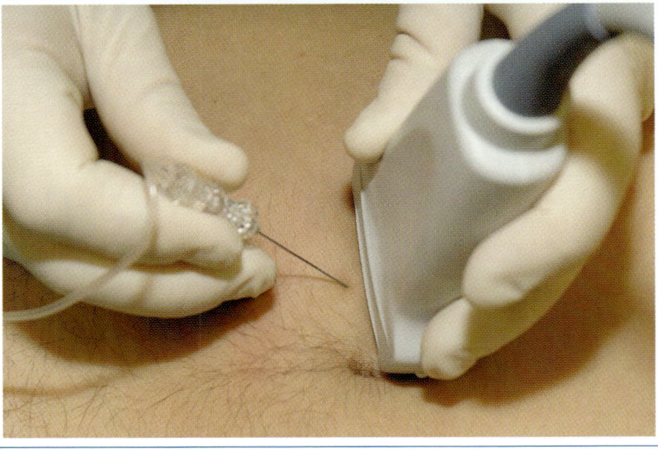

6.2 In-plane needle guidance

In the IP technique, the needle is positioned along the long axis of the ultrasound probe (Figure 6.3). Historically, most peripheral blocks were performed using the IP technique, but in recent years the blocks have been adapted to meet anatomical requirements. The IP technique necessitates that the needle be located inside a 1-mm longitudinal area. Only slight deviations in a lateral direction can cause the needle to disappear from the ultrasound window. Thus, the IP technique needs excellent hand–eye coordination on the part of the physician.

Figure 6.2 Ultrasonographic appearance of the tip of the needle (arrow) when the out-of-plane technique is used

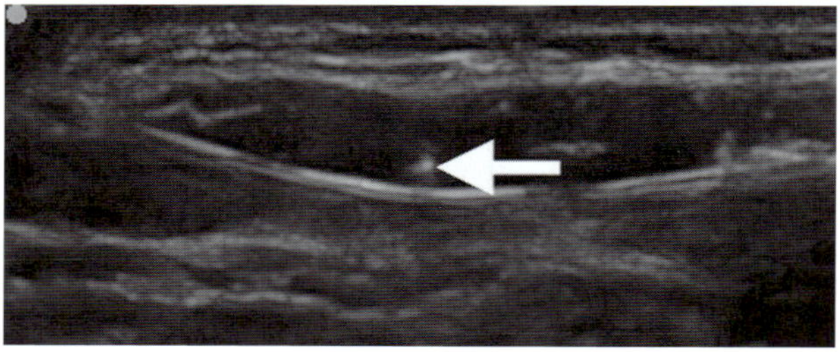

Figure 6.3 In-plane position of the needle relative to the ultrasound probe

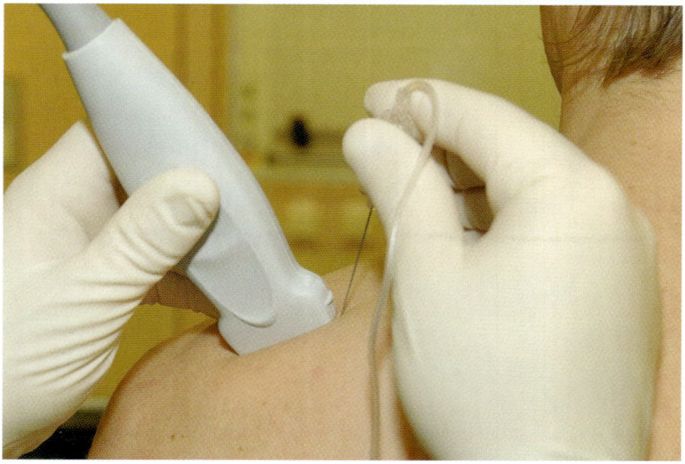

Advancing the needle by the IP technique produces reverberation artefacts and impairs the detection of structures below the body of the needle (Figure 6.4). These artefacts can be avoided by slight lateral movement of the needle (Figure 6.5). In addition, the insertion–target distance is 2–3-fold longer compared with the OOP technique. Nevertheless, we have defined specific indications for the IP technique (e.g., supraclavicular approach to the brachial plexus, popliteal approach to the sciatic nerve, etc.).

Figure 6.4 Ultrasonographic visualization of the body and the tip of the needle when the in-plane technique is used. Reverberation artefacts are clearly visible dorsal to the body of the needle

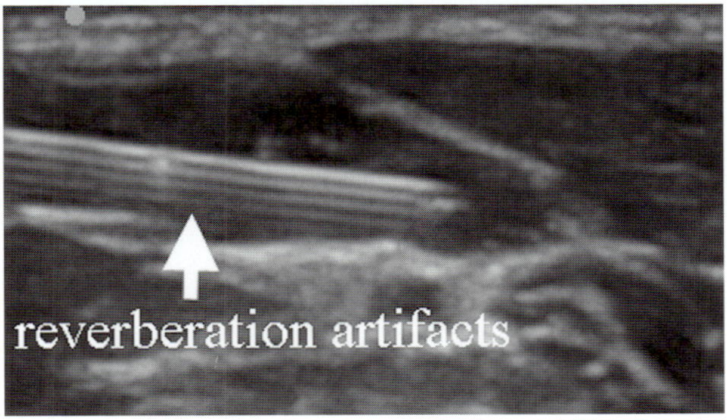

Figure 6.5 Reduced reverberation artefacts during the in-plane technique by lateral movement of the ultrasound probe

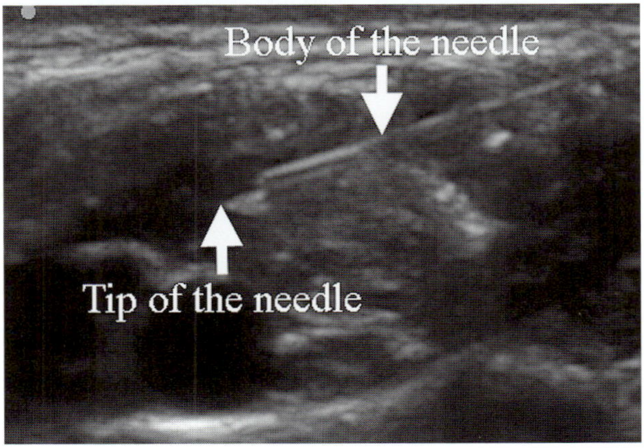

Chapter 7

Pearls and pitfalls

7.1 Setting and orientation of the probe

The position of the anaesthesiologist relative to the patient should be 'face-to-face' with the ultrasound machine positioned lateral to the head of the patient (Figure 7.1). For approaches at the neck, the anaesthesiologist might wish to position themselves behind the head of the patient (Figure 7.2). The orientation of the probe should adhere to a 'true image' (i.e., left side of the probe = left side of the screen).

7.2 Pressure during injection

High-pressure injection of local anaesthetic is associated with neuronal damage and should always be avoided. During performance of specific blocks, for example, an axillary approach to the brachial plexus, where anatomical structures are in close proximity to each other, high-pressure injection can eventually be detected. Where high-pressure injection is detected, the pressure can be alleviated by minimal withdrawal of the needle.

Figure 7.1 'Face-to-face' position of the physician relative to the patient with the ultrasound machine lateral to the head of the patient

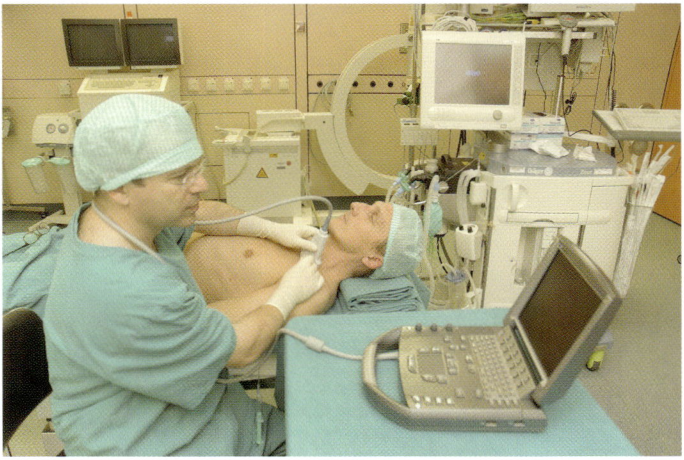

Figure 7.2 Position of the physician behind the patient

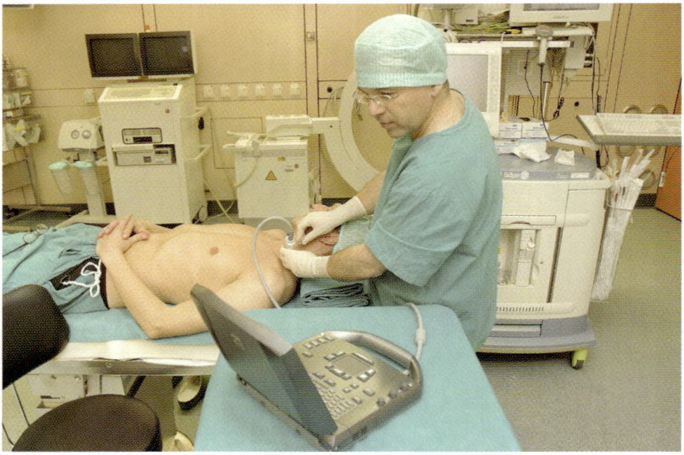

7.3 Extremely superficial structures

For improvement of ultrasonographic visualization of very superficial structures (e.g., superficial branch of the peroneus nerve) a sterile jelly pad may be used to increase the distance from the probe to the skin. A jelly pad also has the advantage that it is totally free of artefacts caused by the traditional application of jelly. This can be important when scanning tiny nerves as even the smallest artefacts may inhibit appropriate visualization of the target structures.

Chapter 8

Neck blocks

8.1 General anatomical considerations

The cervical plexus is formed by the ventral rami of the spinal nerves C1–4. In this context, only the rami of nerves C2–4 are of interest for regional anaesthetic purposes. Each nerve (except the first) divides into an ascending and descending branch to form three communicating loops. The cervical plexus is located at the level of the first four cervical vertebrae, deep beneath the internal jugular vein and anterior to the levator scapulae and middle scalene muscles. The cervical plexus is covered by the sternocleidomastoideus muscle. The branches of the cervical plexus can be classified as either deep or superficial.

8.2 Deep cervical plexus blockade

8.2.1 Anatomy

The deep branches of the cervical plexus can be further subdivided into internal and external series. The internal series is formed by communicating branches consisting of several filaments which pass from the loops between the upper cervical nerves to the vagus and hypoglossus nerves and the sympathetic trunk. Muscular branches supply the longus capitis, rectus capitis lateralis, and anterior muscles. Cervical communicant filaments from the second and third cervical nerves pass downwards to the lateral side of the internal jugular vein, crossing in front of it at the middle of the neck to form a loop with the descending ramus of the hypoglossus nerve (ansa hypoglossi). Another component of the internal series is the phrenic nerve, which mainly arises from the ventral ramus of nerve C4. It passes obliquely on the ventral surface of the anterior scalene muscle, beneath the sternocleidomastoideus and omohyoideus muscles. Finally, it passes between the subclavian vessels and subsequently enters the thorax.

The external series of the deep cervical plexus communicates with the accessory nerve. Muscular branches are distributed to the sternocleidomastoideus, trapezius, levator scapulae, and median scalene muscles.

8.2.1.1 *Anatomical variations*

The anatomical position of the vertebral artery at the level of the upper cervical vertebrae is highly variable. Regardless of this, however, the vertebral artery is in close proximity to the nerve structures. The location of the ansa hypoglossi also varies. It is usually situated between the sternocleidomastoideus muscle and the carotid artery superficial to the internal jugular vein, but it may also be located between the carotid artery and the internal jugular or, in rare cases, dorsal to both vessels. The ansa hypoglossi also varies in length: it may end below the level of the thyroid or at the level of the hyoid bone.

8.2.2 Ultrasound guidance technique

The position of the probe must be strictly lateral at the level of the brachial plexus. Once the C5 root is detected and tracked backwards from the interscalene groove to the transverse process, the probe should be advanced cranially until the C4 root appears. Both the transverse and articular processes have a characteristic contour on ultrasonography. For instance, the nerve root is located at the top of the transverse process (Figure 8.1). The early division of the anterior ramus of the C4 root into a cervical and a brachial branch can usually be detected (Figure 8.2), and similarly for the phrenic nerve. The roots of nerves C2 and C3 can be visualized in an analogue procedure.

Figure 8.1 The C4 root appears (yellow arrow) as a hypoechoic round nerve structure (left side = anterior). AP: articular process; TP: transverse process

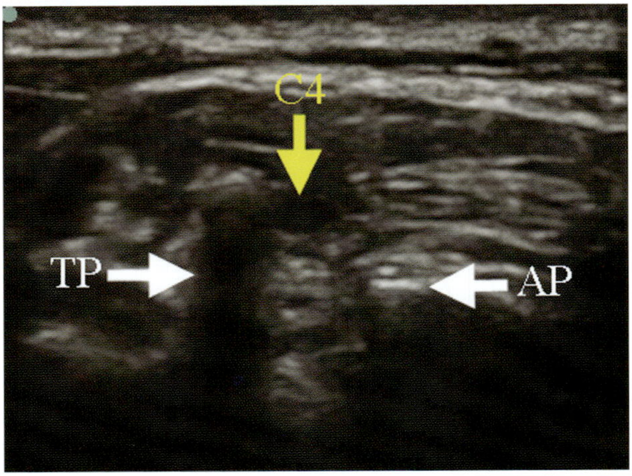

8.2.3 Practical block technique

Once the C4 root is detected at the top of the corresponding transverse process, the block is performed by using the OOP technique with the aim of positioning the tip of the needle dorsal to the root (Figure 8.3). This dorsal block technique has a certain protective effect, avoiding inadvertent slippage of the needle into an artery. The roots of nerves C2 and C3 roots are blocked in an analogue manner.

Figure 8.2 Division of the C4 root into a cervical branch (CB), brachial branch (BB), and the phrenic nerve (PN) (left side = anterior). TP: transverse process

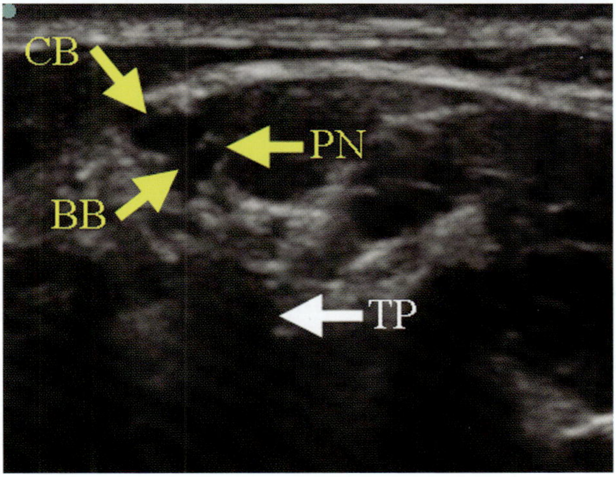

Essentials

Block characteristic	Advanced technique
Patient position	Supine, retroflexed, and slightly contralateral rotated neck
Ultrasound equipment	Linear probe, 25 mm
Specific ultrasound setting	Maximum frequency of the probe
Important anatomical structures	C5 root, transverse and articular processes
Ultrasound appearance of neuronal structures	Hypoechoic, round
Expected Vienna score	2
Needle equipment	50 mm, Facette tip
Technique	OOP
Estimated local anaesthetic volume	2 mL/root

Figure 8.3 Deep cervical plexus blockade. Position of the needle relative to the probe (out-of-plane technique)

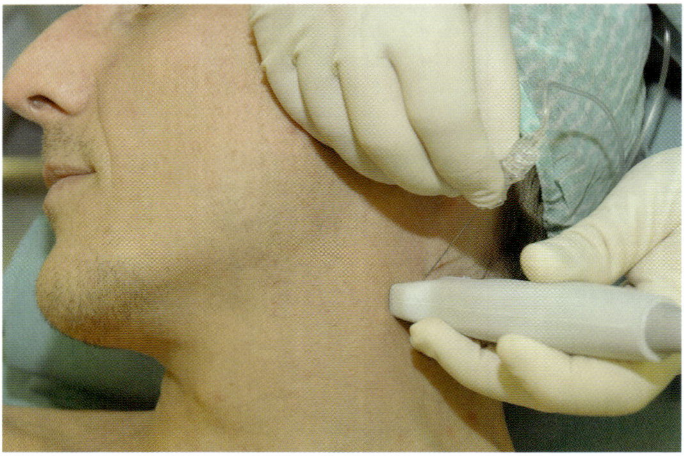

8.3 Superficial cervical plexus blockade

8.3.1 Anatomy

The superficial cervical plexus forms the smaller occipital (from C2), greater auricular (from C2 and C3), cutaneous cervical (from C2 and C3), and supraclavicular (from C3 and C4) nerves.

The smaller occipital nerve curves around and ascends along the posterior border of the sternocleidomastoid muscle, supplies the skin behind the auricula, and communicates with the greater occipital and greater auricular nerves, and the posterior auricular branch of the facial nerve.

The greater auricular nerve winds around the posterior border of the sternocleidomastoid muscle, ascending upon the muscle beneath the platysma to the parotid gland.

The cutaneous cervical nerve turns around the posterior border of the sternocleidomastoid muscle and passes obliquely forward beneath the external jugular vein to the anterior border of the muscle to perforate the deep cervical fascia.

The supraclavicular nerves emerge beneath the posterior border of the sternocleidomastoid muscle, and descends in the posterior triangle of the neck beneath the platysma and deep cervical fascia. Near the clavicle the nerves become cutaneous and arrange into anterior, middle and posterior parts.

8.3.2 Ultrasound guidance technique

The superficial part of the cervical plexus can be visualized between the sternocleidomastoid and levator scapulae muscles, appearing as oval and hyperechoic. An accurate identification of each individual part of the superficial cervical plexus is difficult due to the close proximity of the nerves.

8.3.3 Practical block technique

After identification of the nerve structures between the sternocleidomastoid and levator scapulae muscles at a level slightly above the cricoid cartilage, the block should be performed using an IP technique as illustrated in Figures 8.4 and 8.5. The needle is advanced in the direction of the carotid artery. The spread of local anaesthetic follows the fascial space below the sternocleidomastoid muscle until it reaches the carotic sheath. Ultrasonographic identification of the carotid artery is a prerequisite for safe performance of this technique.

Figure 8.4 Superficial cervical plexus blockade. Position of the needle relative to the probe (in-plane technique)

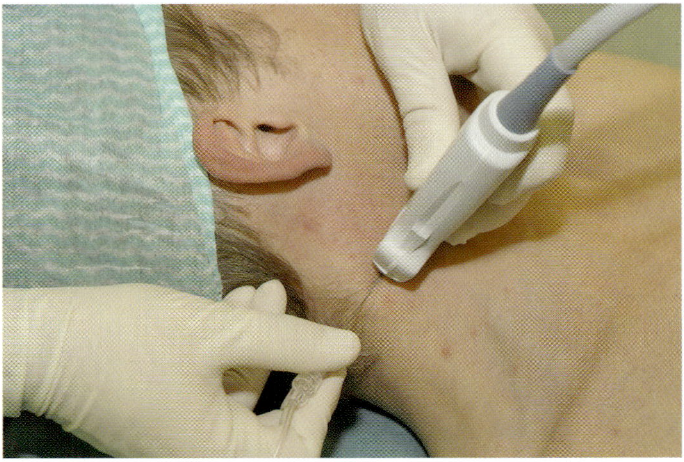

Figure 8.5 Superficial cervical plexus blockade. The local anaesthetic is administered behind the sternocleidomastoid muscle (SCM) in the direction of the carotid artery (CA) (left side = posterior)

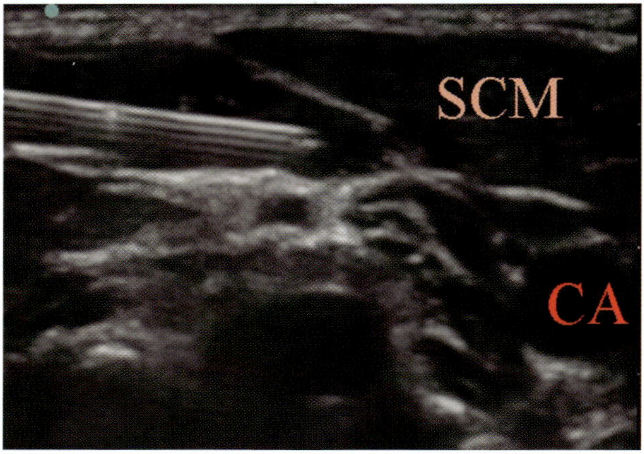

Essentials

Block characteristic	Advanced technique
Patient position	Supine, neck slightly rotated to the contralateral side
Ultrasound equipment	Linear probe, 38 mm
Specific ultrasound setting	Maximum frequency of the probe
Important anatomical structures	Sternocleidomastoid muscle, levator scapulae muscle, carotid artery
Ultrasound appearance of neuronal structures	Hyperechoic, oval
Expected Vienna score	2–3
Needle equipment	50 mm, Facette tip
Technique	IP
Estimated local anaesthetic volume	3–6 mL

Chapter 9

Upper extremity blocks

9.1 General anatomical considerations

The brachial plexus is formed by the ventral rami of the spinal nerves C5–Th1. In general, supraclavicular and infraclavicular parts are described. The ventral rami leave the intervertebral foramina posterior to the vertebral artery and, after a short distance in the scalenovertebral triangle (bordered by the longus colli muscle medially, the anterior scalenus muscle laterally, and the dome of the pleura inferiorly), are situated between the anterior and middle scalene muscles – the interscalene space. The first branches are the dorsal scapular and thoracic longus nerves, both of which pierce the middle scalenus muscle to take a dorsolateral course. Subsequently, the roots form a superior (C5/C6), intermediate (C7), and inferior (C8/T1) trunk.

The third branch in the lateral cervical region is the supraclavicular nerve, which shows a variable level of origin out of the superior trunk. Between the level of the first rib and the clavicle, each trunk bifurcates into an anterior and posterior portion to get rearranged and form the three cords of the brachial plexus. A lateral cord is formed by the anterior portion of the superior and middle trunks, a medial cord by the anterior portion of the inferior trunk, and a posterior cord by the posterior portions of all three trunks. The nomenclature of the three cords (lateral, medial, and posterior) refers to their position around the axillary artery. Note that their respective positions are different in the infraclavicular region (clavipectoral triangle) where they are situated laterally to the artery. The most superficial one is the lateral cord, followed by the posterior and medial cord as the deepest.

The brachial plexus is covered by connective tissue from its origin down to the axillary level. Various septae between the cords and nerves of the plexus appear to be responsible for incomplete nerve blockade, particularly at the axillary level when single-injection techniques are used.

9.2 Interscalene brachial plexus approach

9.2.1 Anatomy

The interscalene groove is bordered by the anterior scalenus muscle medially, the middle scalenus muscle laterally, and the first rib inferiorly. Its location is approximately beneath the lateral border of the sternocleidomastoid muscle when the head is rotated to the opposite side. Of note, the interscalene groove is covered more or less by the sternocleidomastoid muscle in the case of neutral head position. The scalene muscles and the brachial plexus are covered by the praevertebral layer of the cervical fascia. The trunks are formed as described in Section 9.1.

9.2.1.1 *Anatomical variations*

The brachial plexus often receives a communication from the ventral ramus C4. In this case, the plexus is situated more cephalic in relation to the cervical spine and designated as high or *prefixed*. In prefixed plexuses, C4 provides a large branch and the ventral ramus Th1 appears small. When receiving the majority of communications from the ventral ramus C5, the brachial plexus is located more caudally and considered to be low or *postfixed*. In postfixed plexuses, the ventral ramus of Th1 is large, with an additional branch to the plexus provided by Th2.

Variants regarding the course of the brachial plexus and its components have also been described. In a significant number of cases, the nerve roots are located medial (close to the greater vessels of the neck) or lateral to the lateral border of the sternocleidomastoid muscle. The C5 and C6 roots may pierce the anterior scalenus muscle either together or separately. In some cases, only the C5 pierces the anterior scalenus. These situations were found to occur unilaterally or bilaterally to the same extent. In a smaller number of cases, the C5 root may be found completely anterior to the anterior scalenus muscle. A scalenus minimus muscle may be present, visualized as a small muscle slip running anterior to one or two of the roots. In rare cases, the subclavian artery has been found to pierce the anterior scalenus muscle with accompanying post-stenotic dilatation. The dorsal scapular artery (former transversa colli) may arise from the subclavian artery more medially and take an ascending course between the roots. Muscular tissue interposed between the roots is a frequent finding.

9.2.2 Ultrasound guidance technique

The ultrasound investigation starts at the middle of the neck, at the level where the larynx is most prominent and the greater vessels of the neck are easy visible. Thereafter, the probe is moved slowly in a lateral direction until the lateral border of the sternocleidomastoid muscle. Once the lateral border of the sternocleidomastoid muscle and the anterior and middle scalene muscles are depicted, the position of the probe relative to the skin should be slightly moved from a perpendicular in a caudally oblique direction. The nerve roots appear between the anterior and middle scalene muscles inside the posterior interscalene groove as round or oval hypoechoic structures (Figure 9.1).

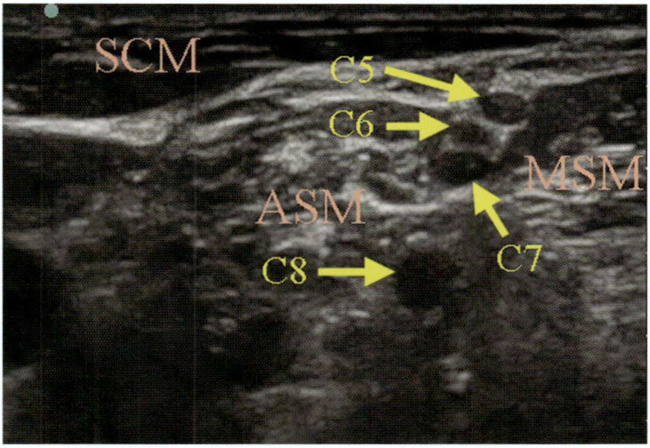

Figure 9.1 Interscalene brachial plexus approach. The hypoechoic nerve roots C5–8 are located between the anterior scalene muscle (ASM) and median scalene muscle (MSM) at the lateral border of the sternocleidomastoid muscle (SCM). A muscle bridge is interposed between the C7 and C8 root (left side = medial).

9.2.3 Practical block technique

It should be taken into consideration that the external jugular vein is usually visible in the final probe position. The puncture site should therefore be chosen medial or lateral to the external jugular vein.

The needle direction relative to the position of the probe should be OOP from cranial (Figure 9.2). Taking a posterior approach using the IP technique can lead to the potential disadvantage of the needle moving perpendicularly to the interscalene groove. As mentioned above, the dorsal scapular and thoracic longus nerves pierce the middle scalenus muscle as first branches of the brachial plexus. They provide motor supply to the shoulder girdle and should be considered at risk if of the IP technique is used in a posterior approach through the middle scalenus muscle. Thus, the OOP technique is the anatomically preferential method. Following positioning of the needle tip between the nerve structures and the middle scalene muscle at the level of the C7 root, the local anaesthetic is administered (Figure 9.3). Depending on the spread of the anaesthetic, redirection of the needle to a position between the nerve structures and the anterior scalene muscle may be necessary. In a minority of cases, the nerve roots will be surrounded following the initial needle position.

If a muscle bridge is detected between the C7 and C8 root, or if blockade of the T1 root is required, it is necessary to adapt the depth of the needle. In these cases, care should be taken to avoid damage of the cervical pleura, for which ultrasound imaging of the cervical pleura is a prerequisite.

Figure 9.2 Interscalene brachial plexus approach. Position of the needle relative to the probe (out-of-plane technique)

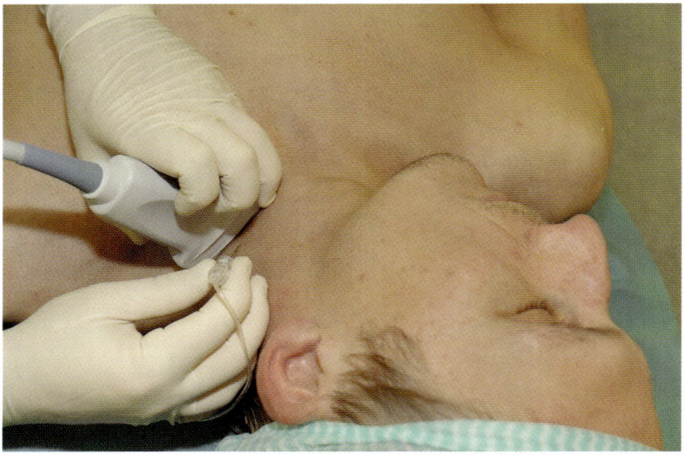

Figure 9.3 Distribution of local anaesthetic (hypoechoic areas indicated by white arrows) around the nerve roots C5–7 (left side = medial). SCM: sternocleidomastoid muscle

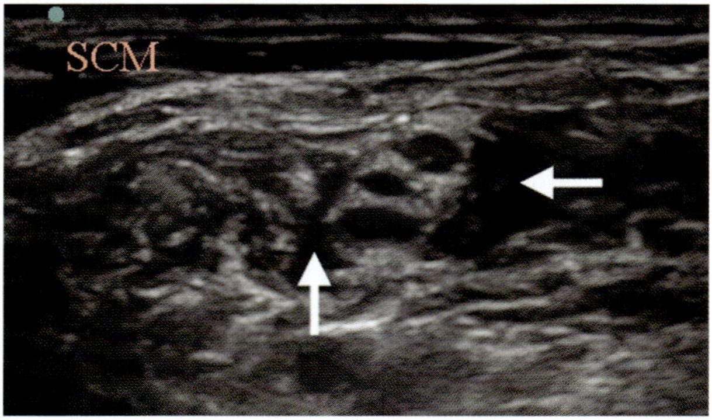

Essentials

Block characteristic	Advanced technique
Patient position	Supine, arm adducted, elbow slightly flexed
Ultrasound equipment	Linear probe, 38 mm
Specific ultrasound setting	Maximum frequency of the probe
Important anatomical structures	Sternocleidomastoid muscle, anterior and middle scalene muscles
Ultrasound appearance of neuronal structures	Round or oval, hypoechoic
Expected Vienna score	1–2
Needle equipment	50 mm, Facette tip
Technique	OOP
Estimated local anaesthetic volume	8–12 mL

Further reading

Kapral S, Greher M, Huber G *et al.* Ultrasonographic guidance improves the success rate of interscalene plexus blockade. *Regional Anaesthesia and Pain Medicine* 2008; **33** (3): 253–8.

9.3 Supraclavicular approach

9.3.1 Anatomy

In the supraclavicular region, between the first rib and the clavicle, the brachial plexus becomes rearranged as described in Section 9.1. The plexus is located laterally to the subclavian artery, which is situated close to the pleura. If present, the dorsal scapular artery (former transverse colli) arises from the subclavian artery and traverses the brachial plexus regularly.

9.3.1.1 *Anatomical variations*

If the dorsal scapular artery has a more prominent appearance than expected, an infraclavicular approach should be considered (see Section 9.4). It should also be noted that the suprascapular nerve has a variable level of origin from the superior trunk.

9.3.2 Ultrasound guidance technique

The ultrasound investigation should start as described for the interscalene approach (Section 9.2.2). Once the brachial plexus is adequately identified within the interscalene space, a further caudal movement of the probe allows the identification of the neural structures as multiple round and oval hypoechoic structures lateral to the subclavian artery (Figure 9.4). The anterior and middle scalene muscles can be traced distally to their insertion on the first rib.

9.3.3 Practical block technique

Once the nerve structures of the brachial plexus and all relevant adjacent anatomical structures (subclavian artery, cervical pleura, and first rib) are identified, an IP technique should be used with a needle insertion site from posterior (Figures 9.5 and 9.6). After careful aspiration and initial administration of a small volume of local anaesthetic, an intermediate analysis of the spread of fluid is mandatory. If the spread is regular, the needle position can be maintained and local anaesthetic should be administered until all nerve structures are surrounded. If the initial needle position does not give a regular spread, the needle should be repositioned. Sometimes a number of needle positions are necessary.

Figure 9.4 Ultrasonographic appearance of the nerve structures of the brachial plexus (yellow arrows) lateral to the subclavian artery (SA) (left side = medial). CP: cervical plexus

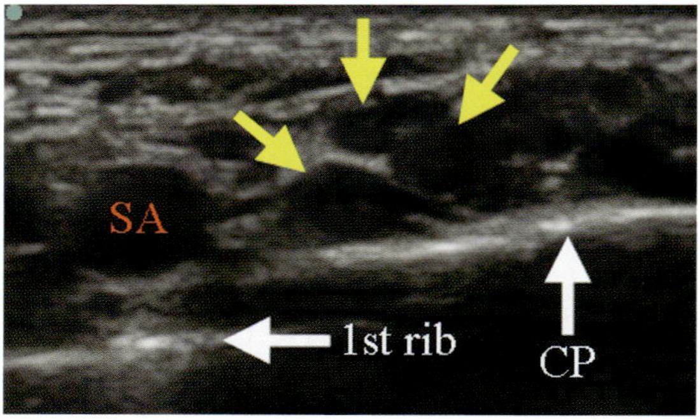

Figure 9.5 Supraclavicular brachial plexus approach. Position of the needle relative to the probe (in-plane technique)

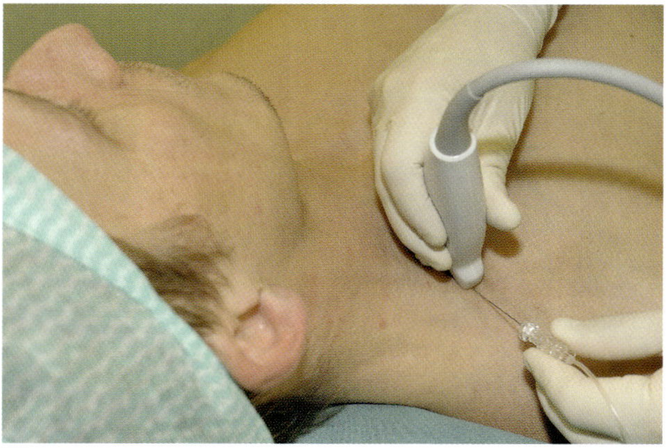

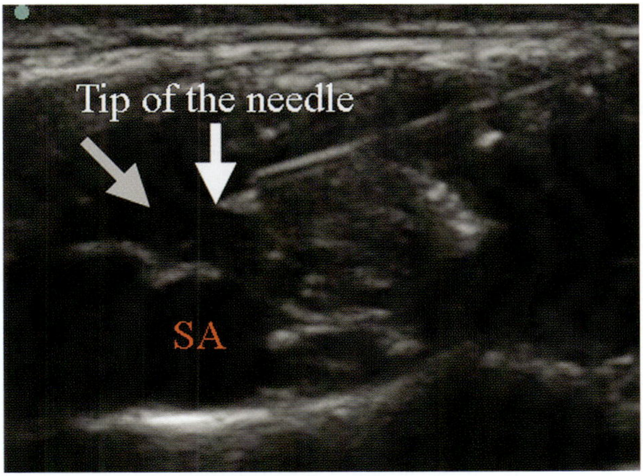

Figure 9.6 Position of the needle above the subclavian artery (SA) and spread of local anaesthetic during supraclavicular brachial plexus blockade (grey arrow = hypoechoic appearance of the local anaesthetic, white arrow = tip of the needle) (left side = medial).

Essentials

Block characteristic	Advanced technique
Patient position	Supine, arm adducted, elbow slightly flexed, neck slightly retroflexed (pillow under shoulders)
Ultrasound equipment	Linear probe, 25 mm
Specific ultrasound setting	Maximum frequency of the probe
Important anatomical structures	Anterior and median scalene muscles, subclavian muscle, subclavian artery, cervical pleura, first rib
Ultrasound appearance of neuronal structures	Round and oval hypoechoic structures
Expected Vienna score	1–2
Needle equipment	50 mm, Facette tip
Technique	IP
Estimated local anaesthetic volume	10 mL

Further reading

Chan V, Perlas A, Rawson R, and Odukoya O. Ultrasound-guided supraclavicular brachial plexus block. *Anesthesia and Analgesia* 2003; **97**: 1514–1517.

Kapral S, Krafft P, Eibenberger K, Fitzgerald A, Gosch M, Weinstabl C. Ultrasound-guided supraclavicular approach for regional anesthesia of the brachial plexus. *Anaesthesia and Analgesia* 1994; **78**: 507–513.

9.4 Infraclavicular approach

9.4.1 Anatomy

The three cords of the brachial plexus (see Section 9.1) enter the infraclavicular region at the clavipectoral triangle lateral to the axillary artery and vein. The cephalic vein, which varies in size, crosses the brachial plexus superficially.

9.4.1.1 *Anatomical variations*

The medial and lateral, or the medial and posterior, cords may be present as a common cord. Rare cases of a single cord have been described. The most common minor variants are related to the position of the cords around the artery.

9.4.2 Ultrasound guidance technique

The position of the ultrasound probe should be 30–45° oblique relative to the clavicle. Using a linear probe at middle frequencies (10 MHz), the subclavian artery is visualized as a round structure and the cords of the brachial plexus as hyperechoic round structures (Figure 9.7). In cases of significant muscle masses above the nerve structures (pectoralis major and minor muscles), optimal visualization of the nerve structures may be impaired. Nevertheless, the medial and lateral cords constantly remain below the fascia of the pectoralis minor muscle. In some cases, an adequate visualization of the posterior cord might be difficult.

Figure 9.7 Ultrasonographic appearance of the cords (yellow arrows) of the brachial plexus lateral to the subclavian artery (SA) (left side = medial). PMM: pectoralis major muscle; white arrow = pleura

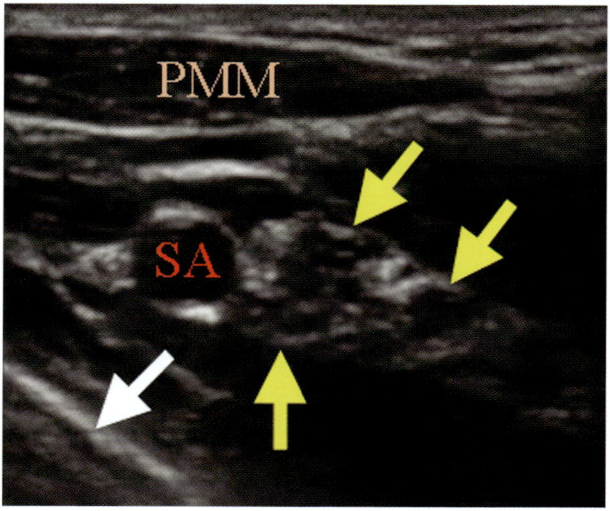

Figure 9.8 Infraclavicular brachial plexus approach. Position of the needle relative to the probe (out-of-plane technique)

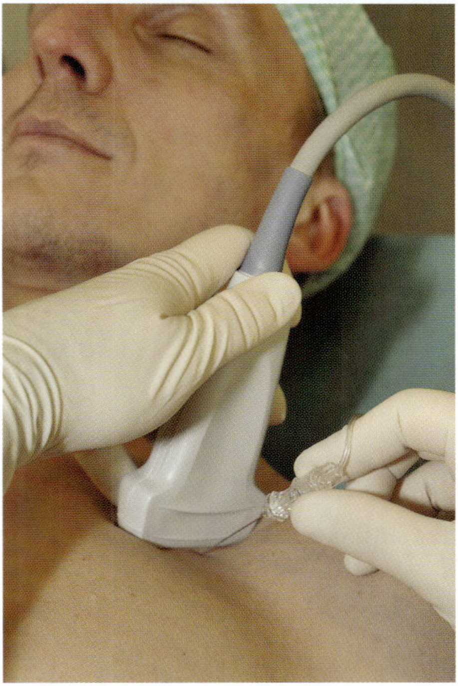

9.4.3 Practical block technique

An OOP technique should be used with a needle position from above or below the probe (Figure 9.8). Once the needle is placed lateral to the subclavian artery and below the pectoralis minor muscle, the local anaesthetic can be administered after careful aspiration. A spread lateral and below the artery provides an optimal block result (Figure 9.9).

Further reading

Sauter A, Smith H, Stubhaug A, Dodgson M, and Klaastad Ø. Use of magnetic resonance imaging to define the anatomical location closest to all three cords of the infraclavicular brachial plexus. *Anesthesia and Analgesia* 2006; **103**: 1574–1576.

Greher M, Retzl G, Niel P, Kamholz L, Marhofer P, and Kapral S. Ultrasonographic assessment of topographic anatomy in volunteers suggests a modification of the infraclavicular vertical brachial plexus block. *British Journal of Anaesthesia* 2002; **88**: 632–636.

Figure 9.9 Spread of local anaesthetic (white arrows) in a lateral direction and below the subclavian artery (SA) (left side = medial)

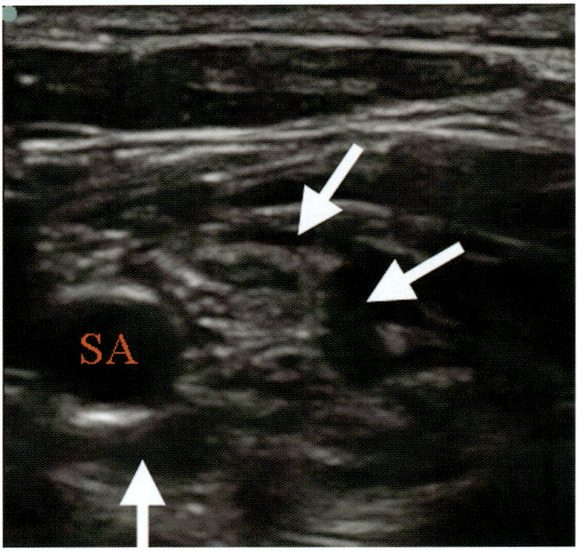

Essentials

Block characteristic	Intermediate technique
Patient position	Supine, arm adducted, elbow slightly flexed
Ultrasound equipment	Linear probe, 38 mm
Specific ultrasound setting	Medium frequency of the probe
Important anatomical structures	Subclavian artery, pectoralis major and minor muscles, pleura
Ultrasound appearance of neuronal structures	Round hyperechoic structures
Expected Vienna score	2–3
Needle equipment	50 mm, Facette tip
Technique	OOP
Estimated local anaesthetic volume	8–15 mL

9.5 Axillary approach

9.5.1 Anatomy

The following anatomical description is based upon a probe position as illustrated in Figure 9.10 where the left side of the image is orientated to the anterior surface of the upper arm. The major branches of the brachial plexus are arranged around the brachial artery in a variable manner. As the most superficial branch, the median nerve is usually found at a 10–12 o'clock position in relation to the artery. The ulnar nerve is usually in a 2–4 o'clock position, but the distance to the artery varies. In a significant number of cases, the basilic vein is interposed between the axillary artery and the ulnar nerve. The radial nerve lies below the artery in a 3–6 o'clock position. The musculocutaneous nerve originates from the lateral cord more proximal at the level of the coracoid process, and usually pierces the coracobrachialis muscle. The medial brachial and medial antebrachial cutaneous nerves are situated superficially beneath the brachial fascia, and their visualization is not always feasible. The brachial artery, together with the median, ulnar, and radial nerves, form a neurovascular bundle that is enveloped by the so-called axillary sheath, which is derived from the prevertebral layer of the cervical fascia. Numerous septae attached to the inner surface of the axillary sheath divide the neurovascular bundle, providing variable compartments for each nerve.

9.5.1.1 *Anatomical variations*

The most frequent variants encountered in the axilla regard the positions of the four nerves around the brachial artery. The site of formation of the median nerve (that is, the union of the medial and lateral branches) has been found as far down as the cubita. The median nerve or its branches may also pass behind the brachial artery.

Figure 9.10 Axillary brachial plexus approach. Position of the needle relative to the probe (out-of-plane technique)

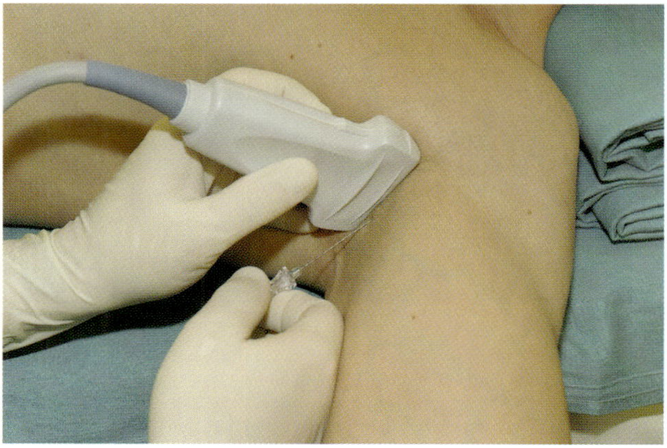

The musculocutaneous nerve typically runs behind the coracobrachialis muscle or between the coracobrachialis muscle and the short biceps head. It frequently occurs that instead of piercing the coracobrachialis muscle, the nerve take a distal course, together with the median nerve, to pass between the biceps and brachialis muscles. Occasionally, only a portion of the nerve follows this course while the main branch pierces the coracobrachialis muscle as usual, subsequently fusing with the aberrant branch. A communicating branch from the median nerve has been described. In some cases the median nerve may be doubled, unusually short, or even absent.

The radial nerve may join the axillary nerve and pass posterior to the humerus. In rare cases, the radial nerve may be absent whereupon the musculocutaneus and ulnar nerves take over its area of supply.

Note that veins may be present in various numbers and diameters.

9.5.2 Ultrasound guidance technique

Due to the fact that all structures in the axilla are in close proximity, it is not always possible to precisely analyse individual nerves using a single and static probe position. Tracking of the nerves facilitates their safe identification. When the axillary artery is scanned from the axillary level in a distal direction, the median nerve is usually found close to the artery. The ulnar nerve can easily be identified as the most superficial nerve and passes beneath the brachial fascia distally to the level of the medial epicondyle. The radial nerve can be tracked from the sulcus of the radial nerve in a proximal direction where it usually lies in a position between the axillary artery and the medial head of the triceps muscle. Figure 9.11 illustrates the location of all three nerves.

By slightly moving the probe from the initial axillary position into a more oblique position, it is possible to visualize the musculocutaneus nerve as a oval hyperechoic structure between the short head of the biceps muscle and the coracobrachial muscle (Figure 9.12). In a more distal position, the form of this nerve appears triangular (Figure 9.13).

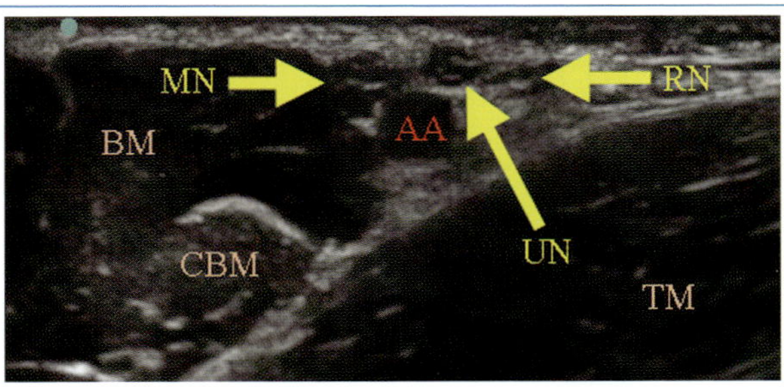

Figure 9.11 Ultrasonographic appearance of the median (MN), ulnar (UN), and radial (RN) nerves around the axillary artery (AA). The MN and UN are in a typical position, while the RN is in a 3 o'clock position relative to the AA. In the majority of cases, the RN is situated below the AA which impairs direct ultrasonographic visualization (left side = cranial). BM: biceps muscle, short head; CBM: coracobrachial muscle; TM: triceps muscle, medial head.

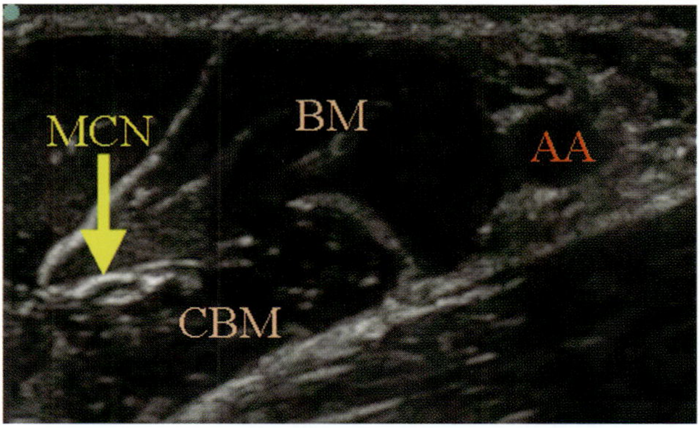

Figure 9.12 Ultrasonographic oval appearance of the musculocutaneus nerve (MCN) between the short head of the biceps (BM) and the coracobrachial muscle (CBM) cranial to the axillary artery (AA) (left side = cranial).

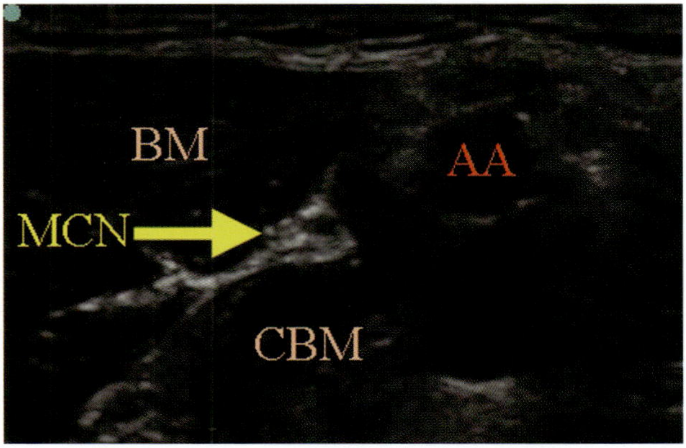

Figure 9.13 Ultrasonographic triangular appearance of the musculocutaneus nerve (MCN) between the short head of the biceps (BM) and the coracobrachial muscles (CBM) cranial to the axillary artery (AA) (left side = anterior).

The probe position described above also enables the location of the axillary nerve (see Figure 9.18). By changing the settings to slightly lower frequencies, the pulsation of the circumflexa humeri posterior artery between the teres major and triceps muscles is possible. The axillary nerve lies in close proximity to that artery.

9.5.3 Practical block technique

After precisely locating the nerves in the axillary region, an OOP technique is indicated for the approach. The needle insertion site should be caudal to the axillary artery in order to avoid muscle puncture. We recommend blocking the deeper structures first and then the more superficial structures. In case of air bubble-related artefacts – which can always occur no matter how well the technique is performed – visibility below the relevant structures is impaired. The radial nerve should therefore be blocked first, followed by the ulnar, median, and musculocutaneus nerves by means of a multi-injection technique (Figures 9.14 and 9.15). Finally, the cutaneous branches of the medial cord should be blocked by administration of a small volume of local anaesthetic beneath the brachial fascia.

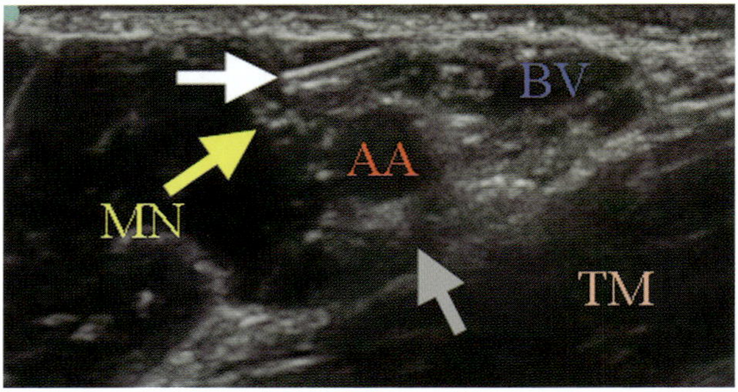

Figure 9.14 Position of the tip of the needle (white arrow) above the median nerve (MN). The hypoechoic area (grey arrow) between the axillary artery (AA) and the triceps muscle (TM) indicates that local anaesthetic has been administered below the axillary artery for blockade of the radial nerve (not directly visible by this ultrasonographic view) (left side = cranial). BV: basilic vein.

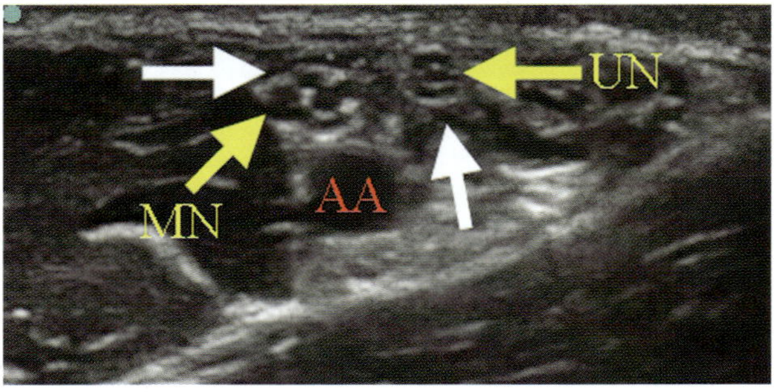

Figure 9.15 The median (MN) and ulnar nerves (UN) surrounded by local anaesthetic (white arrows) (left side = cranial). AA: axillary artery.

Care should be taken to avoid inadvertently positioning the needle intravascularly. If the contact pressure of the ultrasound probe is suboptimal, the veins can disappear from the ultrasound image (Figure 9.16), and intravenous needle position cannot be detected either by direct visualization or by aspiration. The contact pressure of the probe should therefore be carefully adjusted to ensure that vein visibility (Figure 9.17).

Figure 9.16 Axillary artery (AA) during high ultrasound probe contact pressure (left side = cranial)

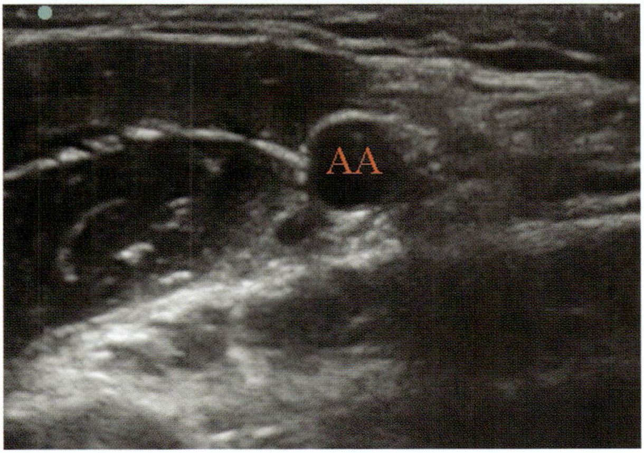

Figure 9.17 Adequate contact pressure of the ultrasound probe (left side = cranial). AA: axillary artery; V: veins

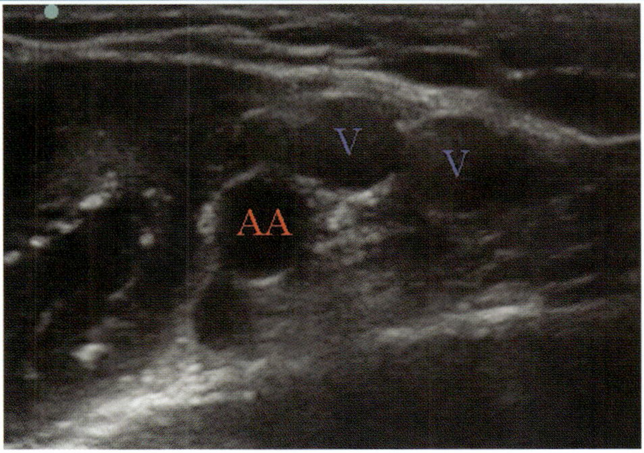

The injection site described above also permits blockade of the axillary nerve, as illustrated in Figure 9.18. Due to the depth of the axillary nerve and the need for lower ultrasound resolution, the nerve is not as clearly visible as the more superficial nerves in that area. Care has to be taken to avoid inadvertent puncture of the circumflexa humeri posterior artery.

Figure 9.18 Ultrasonographic appearance of the axillary nerve (AN) beside the circumflexa humeri posterior artery (CHPA) (left side = cranial)

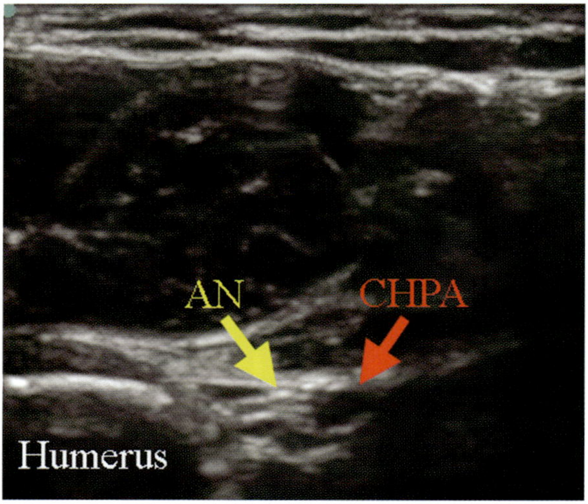

Essentials

Block characteristic	Basic technique
Patient position	Supine, arm 90° abducted
Ultrasound equipment	Linear probe, 38 mm
Specific ultrasound setting	Maximum frequency of the probe
Important anatomical structures	Axillary artery and vein, basilic vein, circumflexa humeri posterior artery (as guidance structure of the axillary nerve), short head of the biceps muscle, coracobrachial muscle, triceps muscle
Ultrasound appearance of neuronal structures	Round and oval hyperechoic structures. The musculocutaneus nerve appears proximal as oval and more distal (between the upper and middle third of the humerus) as triangular hyperechoic structure
Expected Vienna score	1–2
Needle equipment	50 mm, Facette tip
Technique	OOP
Estimated local anaesthetic volume	8–12 mL

Further reading

Retzl G, Kapral S, Greher M, and Mauritz W. Ultrasonographic findings of the axillary part of the brachial plexus. *Anesthesia and Analgesia* 2001; **92**: 1271–1275.

9.6 Suprascapular nerve block

9.6.1 Anatomy

The suprascapular nerve arises from the superior trunk and runs laterally beneath the trapezius and omohyoideus muscles. The nerve enters the supraspinatus fossa through the suprascapular notch below the superior transverse scapular ligament. It gives off branches to the supraspinatus and infraspinatus muscles, and to the shoulder joint.

9.6.1.1 *Anatomical variations*

In some cases, the suprascapular nerve may divide into a superior and inferior branch. The superior branch passes through or above the suprascapular notch, while the inferior branch passes through a foramen below the suprascapular notch. The nerve has also been found to pass over the superior transverse scapular ligament.

9.6.2 Ultrasound guidance technique

With a linear probe positioned in parallel above the spine of the scapula, and following identification of the osseous structure of the notch of the scapula, the suprascapular nerve can be visualized medial to the pulsation of the suprascapular artery (Figure 9.19). Lower frequencies of 8–10 MHz are necessary for optimal visualization of the artery and the nerve. Due to the fact that the nerve may enter the supraspinatus fossa in an oblique direction, its ultrasonographic appearance may be impaired. If this should happen, the angle of the probe should be carefully adjusted both horizontally and vertically until the appearance of the nerve is sufficient. Nevertheless, optimal visualization of the suprascapular nerve may be impaired.

Figure 9.19 Ultrasonographic appearance of the suprascapular nerve (SSN) medial the suprascapular artery (SSA) (left side = medial). SSM: supraspinatus muscle

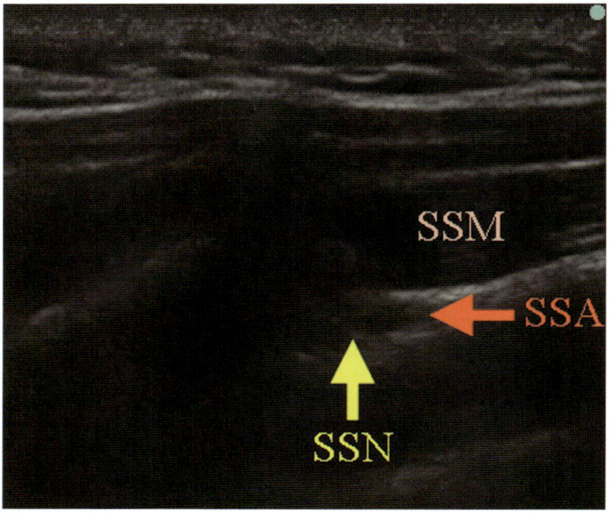

9.6.3 Practical block technique

The block should be performed using an IP technique with the probe in the position as described in Section 9.6.2. The needle insertion site should be medial to the probe (Figure 9.20). It may be difficult to directly visualize the pleura through the notch of the scapula, and if so the needle should not be advanced through the notch. Once the tip of the needle is positioned close to the nerve, negative aspiration prevents inadvertent puncture of the suprascapular artery. A small volume (5 mL) of local anaesthetic usually provides adequate blockade of the suprascapular nerve. A larger volume of local anaesthetic should only be administered in compensation for impaired nerve visualization (as described above).

Figure 9.20 Suprascapular nerve blockade. Position of the needle relative to the probe (in-plane-technique)

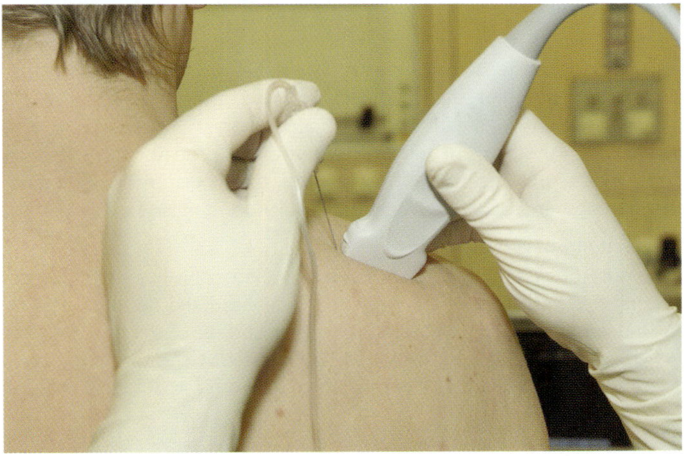

Essentials

Block characteristic	Deeper block, intermediate technique (currently not included in ZUERS recommendations)
Patient position	Sitting, ipsilateral hand lies on contralateral shoulder (increases the distance from the scapula to the posterior thorax wall)
Ultrasound equipment	Linear probe, 25 mm
Specific ultrasound setting	Medium frequency
Important anatomical structures	Notch of the scapula, suprascapular artery
Ultrasound appearance of neuronal structures	Round or oval, slightly hyperechoic
Expected Vienna score	3
Needle equipment	80 mm, Facette tip
Technique	IP
Estimated local anaesthetic volume	5 mL

Further reading

Harmon D and Hearty C. Ultrasound-guided supraclavicular nerve block technique. *Pain Physician* 2007; **10**: 743–746.

9.7 Median nerve block

9.7.1 Anatomy

The median nerve is formed by parts of the lateral and medial cord on the anterior aspect of the brachial artery. It takes its course superficially to the brachial artery to enter the cubital fossa. Here, the nerve is located in a superficial position on the ulnar side of the artery. Subsequently, it usually passes between the humeral and ulnar heads of the pronator teres muscle. At the level of the proximal part of the forearm, the median nerve is embedded between the superficial and profound flexor digitorum muscles.

9.7.1.1 *Anatomical variations*

In a minority of cases, the median nerve may pierce the humeral head of the pronator teres muscle or lie between the ulnar head and the ulna. The nerve has also been found to pass superficially on the surface of the flexor digitorum superficialis muscle. Some reports have observed that the median nerve may split into two branches in the forearm, which pass the carpal tunnel in separate compartments.

9.7.2 Ultrasound guidance technique

The echogenicity of the median nerve at the level of the cubita is moderate. More distal, below the pronator teres muscle, the nerve is hardly visible, whereas at the medial part of the forearm, between the superficial and profound flexor digitorum muscles, it can be visualized clearly as a hyperechoic, round or oval structure (Figure 9.21).

Figure 9.21 Ultrasonographic appearance of the median nerve (MN) between the superficial (SFDM), profound flexor digitorum (PFDM) and flexor pollicis longus (FPLM) muscles (left side = radial)

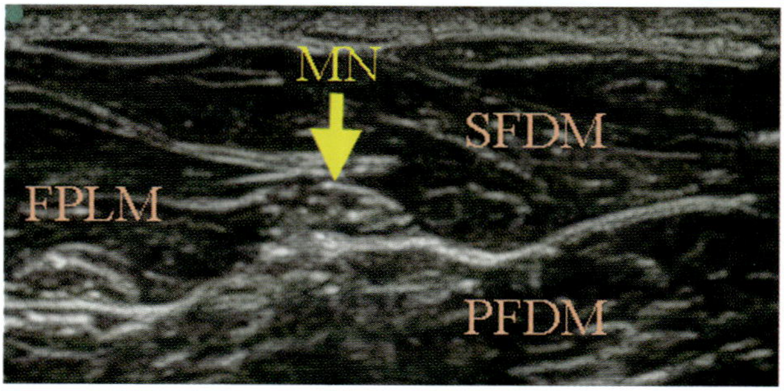

9.7.3 **Practical block technique**

The median nerve should be blocked at the level between the superficial and profound flexor digitorum muscles. More proximal, where the nerve is in close proximity to the brachial artery and several fascial layers, blockade can be difficult due to unpredictable spread of local anaesthetic. Using an OOP technique (Figure 9.22) with the needle between the superficial and profound flexor digitorum muscles at a 6 o'clock position, the nerve can be blocked with small volumes of local anaesthetic (Figure 9.23). When the spread of local anaesthetic is not circumferential, repositioning tip of the needle in a 9 o'clock position and re-administering the drug guarantees a regular blockade.

Figure 9.22 Median nerve blockade. Position of the needle relative to the probe (out-of-plane-technique)

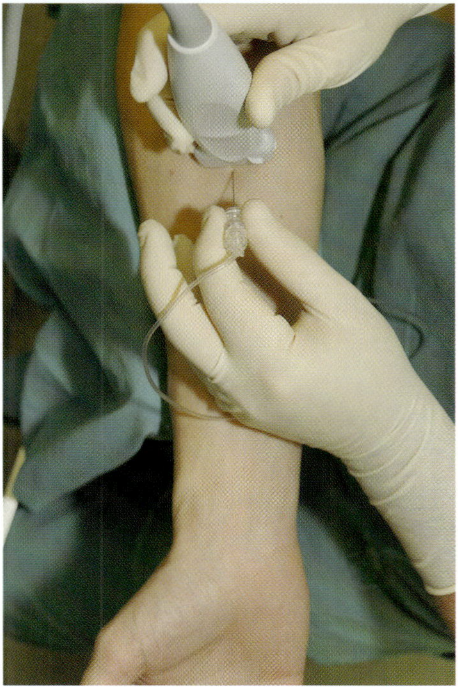

Figure 9.23 **Ultrasonographic appearance of the median nerve (MN) at the forearm after administration of 1.5 mL local anaesthetic (white arrow) (left side = radial)**

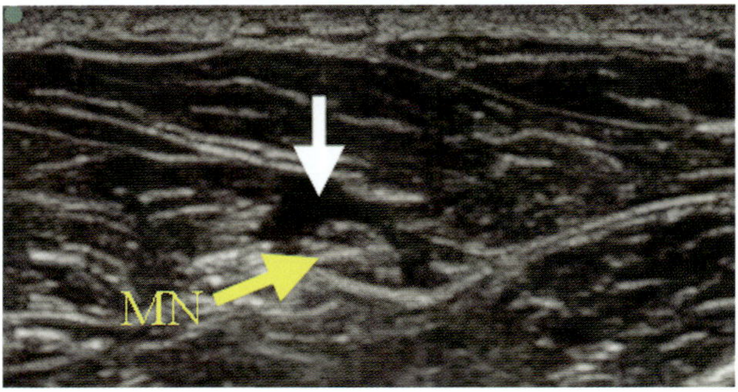

Essentials

Block characteristic	Basic technique
Patient position	Supine, arm slightly abducted, supinated position of the arm
Ultrasound equipment	Linear probe, 25 mm
Specific ultrasound setting	Maximum frequency of the probe
Important anatomical structures	Superficial and profound flexor digitorum muscles
Ultrasound appearance of neuronal structures	Hyperechoic (between the proximal and middle third of the forearm)
Expected Vienna score	1
Needle equipment	50 mm, Facette tip
Technique	OOP
Estimated local anaesthetic volume	2 mL

9.8 Ulnar nerve block

9.8.1 Anatomy

The ulnar nerve is formed by parts of the medial cord and shows a superficial course (subfascial) posterior to the medial intermuscular septum, down to the sulcus of the ulnar nerve on the medial epicondyle of the humerus. Subsequently, the ulnar nerve passes between the two heads of the flexor carpi ulnaris muscle. At the level of the forearm, the nerve is embedded between the flexor carpi ulnar and the superficial and profound flexor digitorum muscles (Figure 9.24). The ulnar artery joins the nerve at a variable level, between the middle and distal third of the forearm (Figure 9.25).

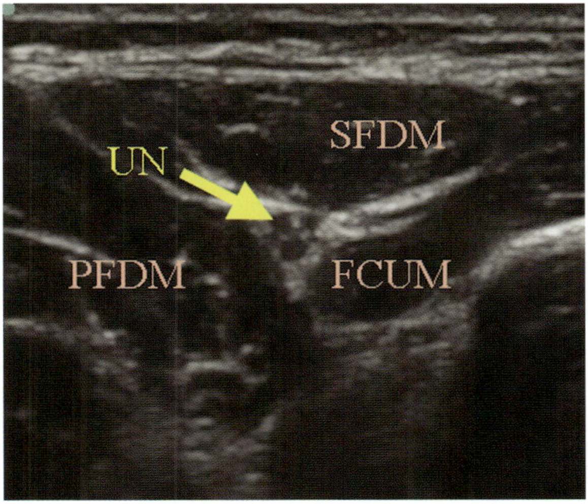

Figure 9.24 Ultrasonographic appearance of the ulnar nerve (UN) at the level of the upper third of the forearm, embedded between the flexor carpi ulnar (FCUM), the superficial (SFDM) and profound flexor digitorum muscles (PFDM) (left side = radial).

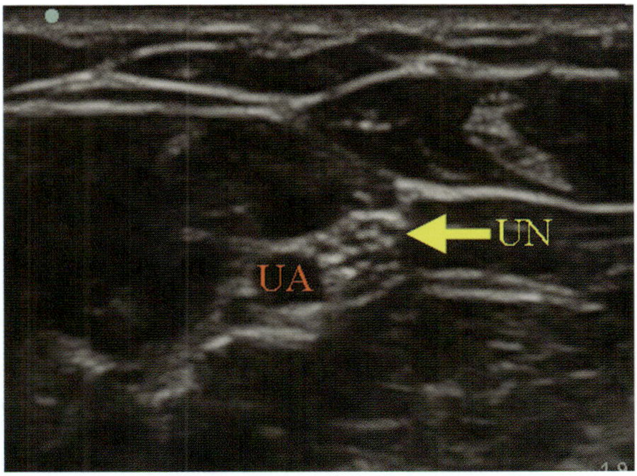

Figure 9.25 Ultrasonographic appearance of the ulnar nerve (UN) at the level of the distal third of the forearm, where the ulnar artery (UA) is in a position radial to the nerve (left side = radial).

9.8.1.1 *Anatomical variations*

In some cases, the ulnar nerve may run anterior to the medial epicondyle of the humerus or lie behind the condyle.

9.8.2 Ultrasound guidance technique

Whereas at the level of the forearm the ulnar nerve appears as a hyperechoic triangular structure (Figure 9.24), above the sulcus of the ulnar nerve it appears as a hyperechoic oval structure (Figure 9.26).

9.8.3 Practical block technique

The ulnar nerve can be blocked above or below the level of the sulcus of the ulnar nerve. Blockade inside the sulcus should always be avoided due the risk of puncture or pressure-related neuronal damage. The optimal position of the block is at the proximal third of the forearm where it is embedded between the flexor carpi ulnar, the superficial flexor digitorum (humeroulnar head), and profound flexor digitorum muscles, and proximal to where the ulnar artery comes in close proximity medial to the ulnar nerve. The preferred block technique is OOP, with the needle direction relative to the probe as illustrated for the median nerve block (see Section 9.7.3). To realize blockade with small amounts of local anaesthetic, two needle positions, first with the tip at the medial and then at the lateral side of the nerve, are required.

Figure 9.26 Ultrasonographic appearance of the ulnar nerve (UN) above the sulcus at the level of the distal third of the upper arm, where the nerve is in a subfascial position (left side = radial)

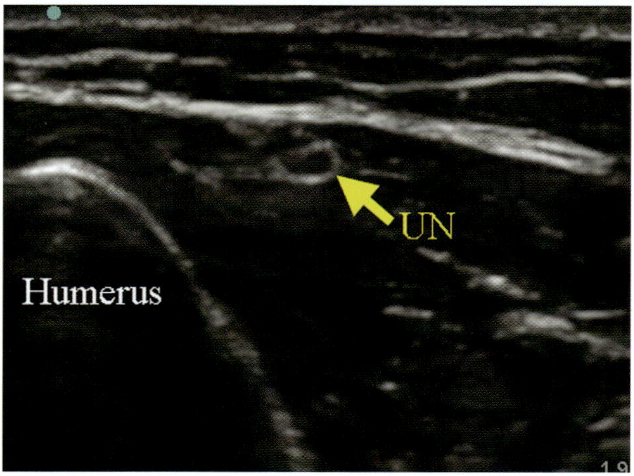

Essentials

Block characteristic	Basic technique
Patient position	Supine, 45° abducted arm, slightly outside rotated
Ultrasound equipment	Linear probe, 25 mm
Specific ultrasound setting	Maximum frequency
Important anatomical structures	Flexor carpi ulnar, superficial flexor digitorum (humeroulnar head), and profound flexor digitorum muscles
Ultrasound appearance of neuronal structures	Hyperechoic, oval (above the sulcus of the ulnar nerve and at the distal third of the forearm) or triangular (at the proximal third of the forearm)
Expected Vienna score	1
Needle equipment	50 mm, Facette tip
Technique	OOP
Estimated local anaesthetic volume	1–2 mL

9.9 Radial nerve block

9.9.1 Anatomy

The radial nerve is formed by the posterior cord. After leaving the axilla, the nerve twists around the dorsal aspect of the humerus in a bony sulcus, accompanied by the profound brachial artery between the medial and lateral heads of the triceps muscle. In the distal third of the upper arm, the radial nerve lies between the brachialis and brachioradialis muscles. The radial nerve reaches the forearm in front of the lateral epicondyle. Here, the radial nerve is usually divided into its superficial and deep branches.

9.9.1.1 *Anatomical variations*

In rare cases, the radial nerve may be absent altogether, whereupon the ulnar and musculocutaneus nerves take over its area of supply. A doubled superficial branch has been observed.

9.9.2 Ultrasound guidance technique

The radial nerve can be visualized proximal to the elbow joint, between the brachialis and coracobrachialis muscles, as a hyperechoic round or slightly oval structure (Figure 9.27). Below the elbow joint, the superficial and profound parts of the radial nerve appear as hyperechoic round structures between the biceps tendon and the brachioradialis muscle (Figure 9.28).

9.9.3 Practical block technique

Blockade of the radial nerve can be performed above or below the elbow joint. From either approach, an OOP technique is recommended with the needle positioned as illustrated for the median nerve block (see Section 9.7.3). If the proximal approach is chosen, a two-injection technique with a needle tip position at the medial and lateral side of the nerve guarantees optimal success.

In cases where the more distal approach is performed, a single injection technique with a needle tip position between the superficial and profound part of the nerve usually provides a sufficient spread of local anaesthetic around the nerve structures.

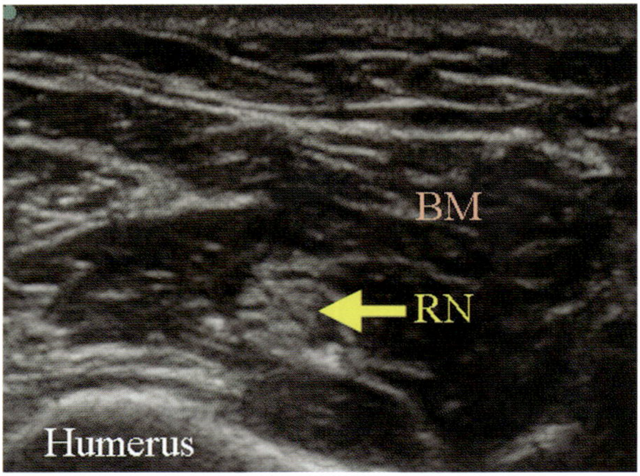

Figure 9.27 Ultrasonographic appearance of the radial nerve (RN) above the elbow (left side = ulnar). BM: brachial muscle.

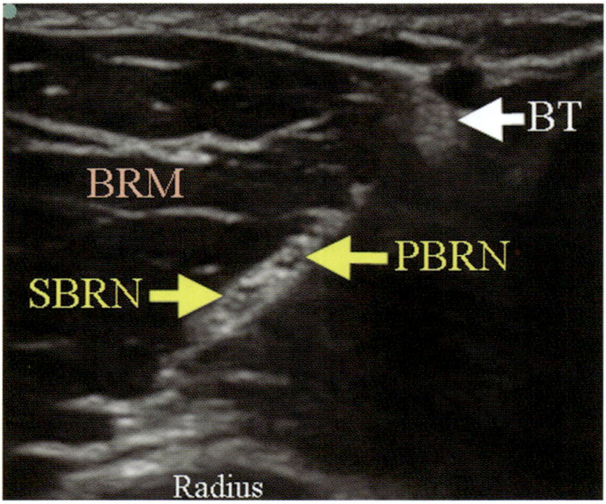

Figure 9.28 Ultrasonographic appearance of the superficial (SBRN) and profound (PBRN) branches of the radial nerve distal to the elbow joint between the biceps tendon (BT) and the brachioradialis muscle (BRM) (left side = radial).

Essentials

Block characteristic	Basic technique
Patient position	Supine, arm slightly abducted
Ultrasound equipment	Linear probe, 25 mm
Specific ultrasound setting	Maximum frequency
Important anatomical structures	Above the elbow: brachial muscle Below the elbow: brachioradialis muscle and biceps tendon
Ultrasound appearance of neuronal structures	Above the elbow joint: hyperechoic, round or slightly oval Below the elbow joint: hyperechoic, round
Expected Vienna score	1–2
Needle equipment	50 mm, Facette tip
Technique	OOP
Estimated local anaesthetic volume	2–3 mL

Further reading

McCartney C, Xu D, Constantinescu C, Abbas S, and Chan V. Ultrasound examination of peripheral nerves in the forearm. *Regional Anesthesia and Pain Medicine* 2007; **32**: 434–439.

Chapter 10

Lower extremity blocks

10.1 General anatomical considerations

The *lumbar plexus* derives from the ventral rami of the spinal nerves L1–L3 and parts of L4 (furcal nerve). The first lumbar ramus commonly receives a branch from Th12. The lumbar plexus is formed within the posterior portion of the psoas major muscle. The branches of the lumbar plexus are the iliohypogastric, ilioinguinal, genitofemoral, femoral, lateral femoral cutaneous, and obturator nerves.

The *sacral plexus* is formed by parts of the ventral rami L4 and L5 (lumbosacral trunk) together with the ventral rami of the sacral nerves S1–S3. The sacral plexus is located within the pelvis on the ventral surface of the piriformis muscle. The major branches relevant for regional anaesthesia are the sciatic and posterior femoral cutaneous nerves. Due to its location within the pelvis, the sacral plexus cannot be accessed.

10.2 Psoas compartment block

10.2.1 Anatomy

The term 'psoas compartment block' was introduced decades ago to describe a potential space between the psoas major and quadratus lumborum muscles. However, several anatomical studies have since demonstrated that the lumbar plexus is located within the substance of the psoas major muscle. Therefore, the term 'psoas compartment' should be used to describe the layer within the muscle which contains the lumbar plexus and its branches. The iliohypogastric and ilioinguinal nerves emerge from the upper lateral border of the psoas muscle, whereas the genitofemoral nerve leaves the muscle on its ventral surface. The femoral nerve exits the muscle on its posterolateral surface to lay in the gutter between the psoas major und iliacus muscles. The lateral femoral cutaneous nerve emerges from the lateral border of the psoas muscle. In contrast, the obturator nerve descends within the muscle and emerges from its posteromedial border. At the level L4–5, the main nerves of the lumbar plexus (femoral, obturator, and lateral femoral cutaneous) are situated within the posterior part of the psoas major muscle in the vast majority of patients. Here, they can be accessed by a posterior approach.

10.2.1.1 *Anatomical variations*

The lumbar plexus may be also encountered in high (prefixed) or low (postfixed) form. Whereas in the prefixed form, the plexus receives a branch from T12, in the postfixed form the ventral ramus L5 contributes to the plexus. In rare cases, the entire plexus is located posterior to the psoas major muscle, adjacent to the lumbar transverse processes. This variant should be considered when nerve stimulation fails to locate the plexus within the psoas muscle. Additionally, the femoral nerve shows a remarkable degree of branching within the psoas muscle in some cases. Two or three branches of the femoral nerve may be found within the psoas major muscle. This might explain partial block effects since the respective branches are separated by more or less muscular tissue.

10.2.2 **Ultrasound guidance technique**

Ultrasonography of the lumbar paravertebral region provides reliable and detailed imaging of the psoas major muscle and the surrounding structures. Curved array transducers operating at lower frequencies were found to be the best choice for this purpose. Due to the deep location of the lumbar plexus and the typical echo texture of the psoas major muscle, delineation of neural structures is difficult in the adult population since the distance between the skin and the plexus increases with body mass index. Thus, we recommend the additional use of nerve stimulation to help locate the lumbar plexus.

Patient positioning is equivalent to the classic technique: lateral decubitus position with the operated side uppermost, hips and knees slightly flexed. Identifying the lumbar levels can be best achieved by means of a longitudinal paravertebral sonogram showing the lumbar transverse processes. They can be counted in a cephalic direction, beginning at the posterior surface of the sacrum. The L4/L5 transverse processes, and subsequently the intertransverse space, should be identified. The transducer should then be rotated into a transverse plane to delineate the psoas major muscle at the intertransverse space. Best imaging of the entire paravertebral region is achieved with a transducer position 5–6 cm lateral from the spinous processes. Here, the muscle has an oval-shaped configuration with an echo texture typically consisting of hyperechoic striations on a hypoechoic background. The hyperechoic structures correspond to tendon-like bundles of fibrous tissue within the muscle that can be misinterpreted as neural structures.

The adjacent structures are the lower pole of the respective kidney laterally (may descend down to L4, especially during deep inspiration), the adjacent vertebral body medially, the erector spinae muscle dorsally, and the retroperitoneal space ventrally. The quadratus lumborum muscle is situated posterolateral to the psoas major muscle (Figure 10.1).

10.2.3 **Practical block technique**

After identifying the relevant structures at the L4–5 level, both a skin and a deep subcutaneous infiltration should be performed close to the medial side of the transducer. A 100–150 mm long needle is inserted using the IP technique (Figure 10.2). The needle is gently advanced through the erector spinae to access

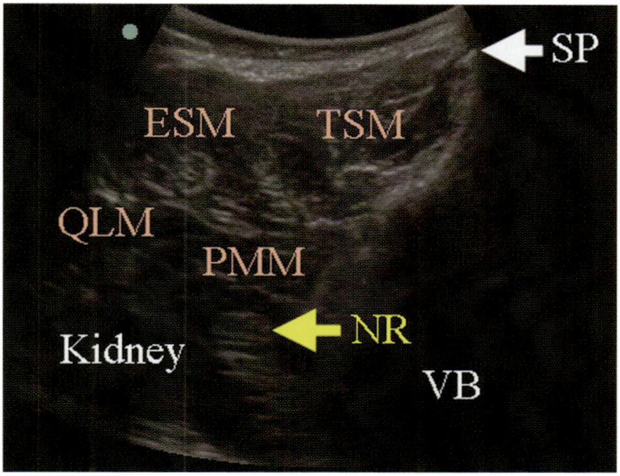

Figure 10.1 Ultrasonographic illustration of the lumbar paravertebral region at the L3/4 level. The position of the nerve root can be estimated between the posterior and middle third in cases when the nerve structures are not directly visible (left side = lateral). ESM: erector spinae muscle; NR: nerve root; PMM: psoas major muscle; QLM: quadratus lumborum muscle; SP: spinous process; TSM: transversospinal muscle; VB: vertebral body.

Figure 10.2 Psoas compartment blockade. Position of the needle relative to the probe (in-plane-technique)

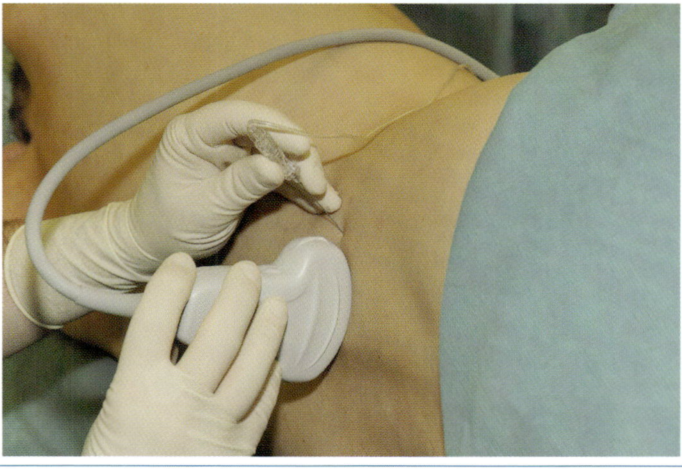

Essentials

Block characteristic	Advanced technique
Patient position	Lateral position with the operated side uppermost, hips and knees slightly flexed
Ultrasound equipment	Curved array probe
Specific ultrasound setting	Low frequency, choose 'abdominal' preset
Important anatomical structures	Psoas major, quadratus lumborum, and erector spinae muscles, vertebral body, kidney
Ultrasound appearance of neuronal structures	–
Expected Vienna score	4
Needle equipment	80–150 mm, Facette tip
Technique	IP
Estimated local anaesthetic volume	20 mL

the posterior part of the psoas major muscle. Piercing the inner layer of the thoracolumbal fascia can be felt as a clear pop and occasionally provokes a painful sensation.

In most cases, the lumbar plexus is located within the posterior part of the psoas major muscle. Using a nerve stimulator, twitches of the quadriceps muscle are commonly obtained at a depth of 6–9 cm, depending on body mass index. A stimulation threshold of 0.4–0.5 mA is satisfactory. Twitches of the adductor muscles indicate a medial needle position that should be corrected as epidural spread of local anaesthetic is possible. Although the correct needle position should be confirmed by ultrasound imaging, an initial test dose can be recommended to rule out intrathecal spread in cases of uncertainty. After careful aspiration, the local anaesthetic solution should be injected in fractions to detect acute systemic toxicity, since false-negative aspiration tests are possible. Injection of local anaesthetic solution causes a diffuse distension of the psoas major muscle in contrast to superficial blocks, where a distinct volume effect is recognized. A total volume of 25 mL local anaesthetic solution usually provides a sufficient block of the main branches of the lumbar plexus.

Suggested Literature

Ultrasound Guidance for the Psoas Compartment Block: An Imaging Study. Kirchmair L, Entner T, Kapral S, Mitterschiffthaler G. *Anaesthesia Analgesia* 2002; **94**(3): 706–710.

10.3 Femoral nerve block

10.3.1 Anatomy

The femoral nerve as the largest branch of the lumbar plexus arises from the ventral rami L1-4. It passes distally between psoas major and iliacus muscles to reach the lacuna musculorum. At this site the femoral nerve is located beneath the inguinal ligament, lateral to the femoral vessels and on the anterior surface of the iliopsoas muscle covered by its fascia. Subsequently, the nerve divides into several branches: an anterior group for sensory supply, a medial and lateral group for motor supply.

10.3.1.1 *Anatomical variations*

The femoral nerve may arise from T12-L4 (prefixed plexus) or L1-5 (postfixed plexus). Instead of running on the anterior surface of the iliopsoas muscle the nerve may pierce the latter. The nerve was also found between the femoral vessels.

10.3.2 Ultrasound guidance technique

Using a high-frequency linear probe, the nerve should be located above or slightly distal to the inguinal ligament. The nerve itself appears less echoic on ultrasonography than other nerves (Figure 10.3) and is located in a very close position relative to the psoas major muscle.

Figure 10.3 Ultrasonographic appearance of the femoral nerve (FN) slightly distal the inguinal ligament and lateral the femoral artery (FA) (left side = medial). IPA: iliopectineal arch; IPM: iliopsoas muscle

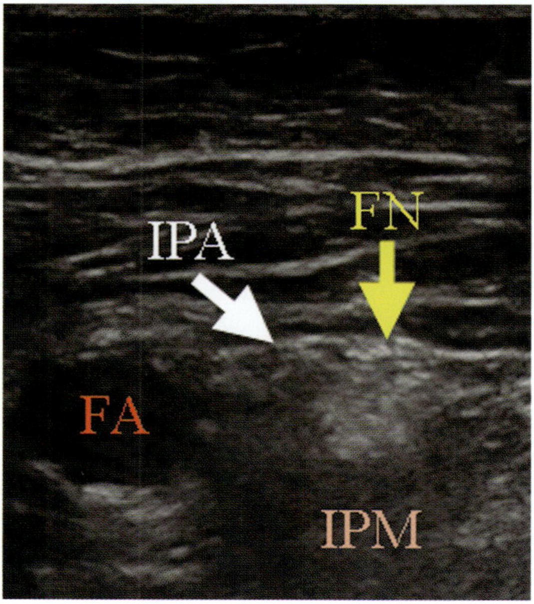

10.3.3 Practical block technique

Since the femoral nerve divides slightly distal to the inguinal ligament in several branches, blockade should be performed as proximal as possible, but always below the inguinal ligament. As described above, the poor echogenicity of the femoral nerve may make it difficult to visualize. Therefore, careful probe adjustments should be performed to optimize the visibility of the nerve. The large femoral vessels serve as clear guidance structures. The OOP needle direction is the preferred technique for this block (Figure 10.4). Because the nerve is embedded in muscle structures, the local anaesthetic should be administered carefully in order to avoid intraneuronal injection.

Essentials

Block characteristic	Basic technique
Patient position	Supine, slightly outside rotated lower extremity
Ultrasound equipment	Linear probe, 38 mm
Specific ultrasound setting	Maximum frequency
Important anatomical structures	Femoral artery, iliopectineal arch, iliopsoas muscle
Ultrasound appearance of neuronal structures	Poor echogenicity, round to oval
Expected Vienna score	2–3
Needle equipment	50 mm, Facette tip
Technique	OOP
Estimated local anaesthetic volume	5 mL

Figure 10.4 Femoral nerve blockade. Position of the needle relative to the probe (out-of-plane technique)

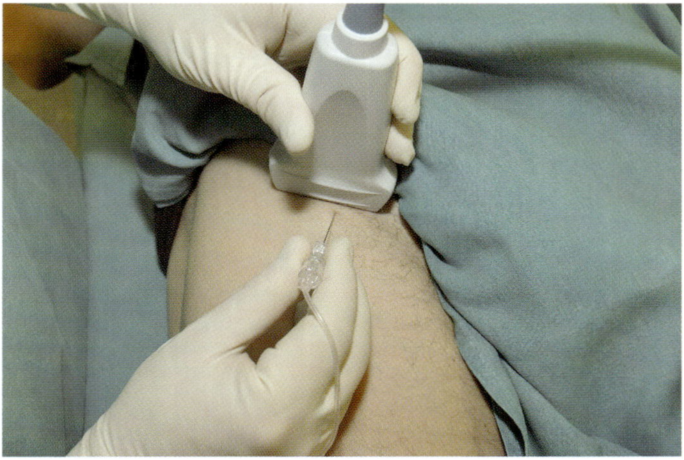

Further reading

Marhofer P, Schrögendorfer K, Koinig H, Kapral S, Weinstabl C, and Mayer N. Ultrasonographic guidance improves sensory block and onset time of three-in-one blocks. *Anesthesia and Analgesia* 1997; **85**: 854–857.

Marhofer P, Schrögendorfer K, Wallner T, Koinig H, Mayer N, and Kapral S. Ultrasonographic guidance reduces the amount of local anaesthetic for 3-in-1 blocks. *Regional Anesthesia and Pain Medicine* 1998; **23**: 584–588.

10.4 Saphenous nerve block

10.4.1 Anatomy

The saphenous nerve is a pure sensory branch of the femoral nerve. It lies inside the adductor canal in front of the femoral artery down to the lower part of the adductor magnus muscle, where the nerve separates from the artery to descend vertically to the medial side of the knee behind the sartorius muscle. After piercing the fascia lata, the nerve lies between the tendons of the gracilis and sartorius muscles and becomes subcutaneous. Infrapatellar branches of the saphenous nerve supply a skin area distal to the patella. At the tibial side of the leg, the saphenous nerve is accompanied by the great saphenous vein.

10.4.1.1 *Anatomical variations*

In some cases, the saphenous nerve may pierce the sartorius muscle. It has also been found to terminate at the level of the knee joint. A branch of the tibial nerve may then cover its area of supply. The infrapatellar branch may originate from the branch to the vastus medialis muscle and may pierce, pass superficially, or pass beneath the sartorius muscle.

10.4.2 Ultrasound guidance technique

The femoral artery is visualized at the medial side of the thigh. Where the artery is situated deeply, colour Doppler scanning might be useful. The saphenous nerve is located above the artery and appears there as a hyperechoic round structure (Figure 10.5). Tracking the nerve and artery in a distal direction shows that the femoral artery descends down the adductor canal, whereas the nerve moves in a more superficial position behind the sartorius muscle (Figure 10.6).

10.4.3 Practical block technique

Once the saphenous nerve is identified behind the sartorius muscle as a hyperechoic round structure, the block can be performed using the IP technique (Figure 10.7). The needle should be guided carefully behind the sartorius muscle until the nerve is approached.

More distal and anterior to the medial malleolus, the nerve can be blocked using the OOP technique. The probe should be placed with minimal pressure in order to avoid compression of the great saphenous vein, which carries the risk of inadvertently and unknowingly positioning the needle tip intravascularly.

Figure 10.5 Ultrasonographic appearance of the saphenous nerve (SN) in a 12 o'clock position relative to the femoral artery (FA) (left side = caudal). SM: sartorius muscle

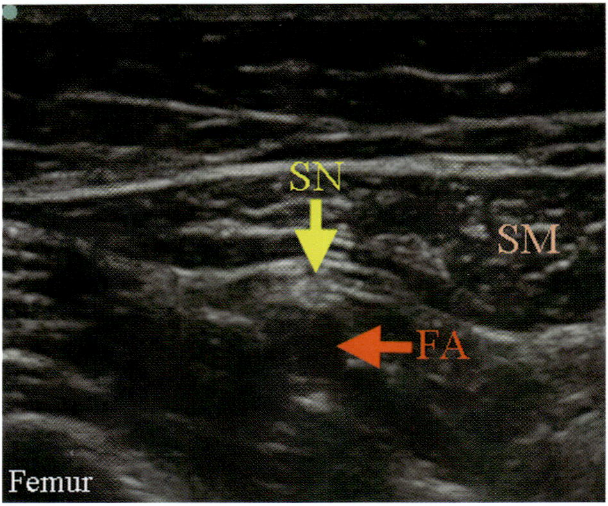

Figure 10.6 Ultrasonographic appearance of the saphenus nerve (SN) behind the sartorius muscle (SM) in a more distal position as illustrated in figure 90. (left side = caudal)

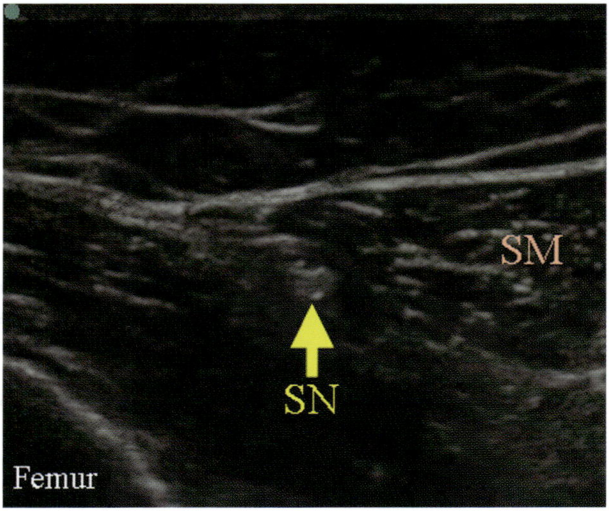

Figure 10.7 Saphenous nerve blockade. Position of the needle relative to the probe (in-plane technique)

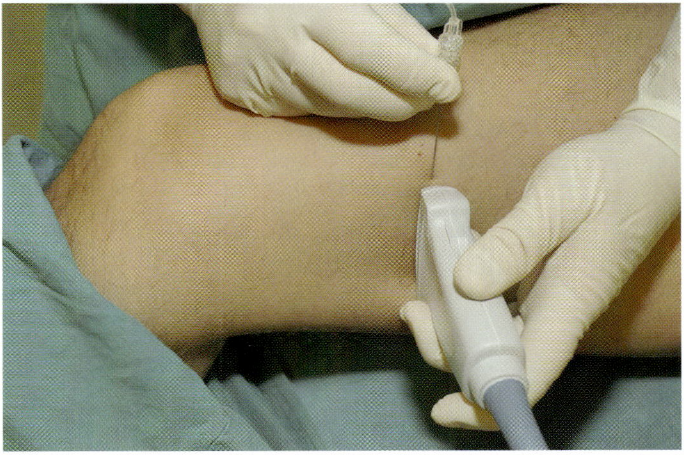

Essentials

Block characteristic	Basic technique
Patient position	Supine, slightly outside rotated lower leg and slightly flexed knee
Ultrasound equipment	Linear probe
Specific ultrasound setting	Medium frequency when the femoral artery in visualized, high frequency during tracking of the saphenous nerve
Important anatomical structures	Femoral artery, sartorius muscle
Ultrasound appearance of neuronal structures	Hyperechoic, round
Expected Vienna score	1–2
Needle equipment	50 mm, Facette tip
Technique	Proximal: IP Distal: OOP
Estimated local anaesthetic volume	Proximal: 2–3 mL Distal: 1–2 mL

10.5 Blockade of the infrapatellar branch

10.5.1 Anatomy

At the level of the knee the saphenous nerve gives off a large infrapatellar branch, which pierces the sartorius muscle and the fascia lata to supply the skin in front of the patella. The infrapatellar branch later forms the plexus patellae, together with branches of the lateral cutaneous femoral nerve.

10.5.2 Ultrasound guidance technique

Once the saphenous nerve is detected below the sartorius muscle, the infrapatellar branch can be visualized as a hyperechoic round structure located more superficially below the sartorius muscle compared with the saphenous nerve (Figure 10.8). Tracking the branch more distally, it is possible to detect piercing of the sartorius muscle.

10.5.3 Practical block technique

The infrapatellar branch can be blocked slightly distal to the described site of blockade for the saphenous nerve using an IP technique. The technique itself is exactly the same as described for the saphenous nerve (see Section 10.4.3).

Essentials

Block characteristic	Basic technique
Patient position	Supine, slightly outside rotated lower leg and slightly flexed knee
Ultrasound equipment	Linear probe
Specific ultrasound setting	High frequency
Important anatomical structures	Saphenous nerve, sartorius muscle
Ultrasound appearance of neuronal structures	Round, hyperechoic
Expected Vienna score	2
Needle equipment	50 mm, Facette tip
Technique	IP
Estimated local anaesthetic volume	2 mL

Figure 10.8 Ultrasonographic appearance of one infrapatellar branch (IB) (left side = caudal). SM: sartorius muscle

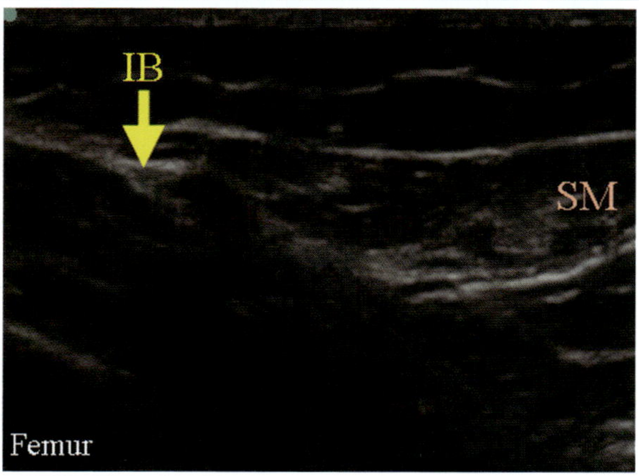

Further reading

Lundblad M, Kapral S, Marhofer P, and Lönnqvist PA. Ultrasound-guided infrapatellar nerve block in human volunteers: description of a novel technique. *British Journal of Anaesthesia* 2006; **97**: 710–714.

10.6 Lateral cutaneous femoral nerve block

10.6.1 Anatomy

The lateral femoral cutaneous nerve usually arises from the ventral rami L2–3. It crosses the iliacus muscle obliquely toward the anterior superior iliac spine, where it passes medially to the latter below the inguinal ligament, over the sartorius muscle and into the thigh.

10.2.1.1 *Anatomical variations*

The lateral femoral cutaneous nerve may arise from L1–2 (prefixed plexus) or from L3–4 (postfixed plexus). It may be missing on one side and be replaced by an anterior cutaneous branch of the femoral nerve or by the ilioinguinal nerve. The nerve may pass beneath the inguinal ligament more medially (between the anterior superior iliac spine and the femoral vessels). It may pierce, pass anterior to, or pass posterior to the sartorius muscle.

10.6.2 Ultrasound guidance technique

The lateral cutaneous femoral nerve is in a position closely medial to the anterior superior iliac spine, and above, inside, or posterior the sartorius muscle. Since the sartorius muscle originates from the anterior superior iliac spine, the hyperechoic appearance of the tendon of the muscle impairs the visibility of the hyperechoic nerve. Improved visibility may be achieved with a slightly more distal position of the probe. The nerve itself should appear as a hyperechoic round structure above the belly of the sartorius muscle (Figure 10.9).

Figure 10.9 Ultrasonographic appearance of the lateral cutaneous femoral nerve (LCFN) slightly medial to the anterior superior iliac spine (right to the nerve) (left side = medial). SM: sartorius muscle

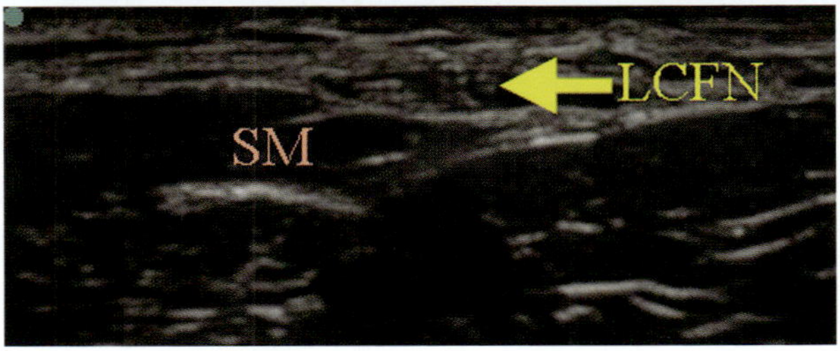

10.6.3 Practical block technique

Following administration of larger volumes of local anaesthetics (20 mL) during femoral nerve blockade, an additional block of the lateral cutaneous femoral nerve can be achieved. When a single blockade of the lateral cutaneous femoral nerve is indicated, the nerve should be visualized medial and slightly caudal to the anterior superior iliac spine, above the belly of the sartorius muscle, using the OOP technique with a needle position below the probe (Figure 10.10).

Essentials

Block characteristic	Basic technique
Patient position	Supine
Ultrasound equipment	Linear probe
Specific ultrasound setting	High frequency
Important anatomical structures	Anterior superior iliac spine, sartorius muscle, inguinal ligament
Ultrasound appearance of neuronal structures	Hyperechoic, round
Expected Vienna score	2
Needle equipment	50 mm, Facette tip
Technique	OOP
Estimated local anaesthetic volume	1–2 mL

Figure 10.10 Lateral cutaneous femoral nerve blockade. Position of the needle relative to the probe (out-of-plane technique)

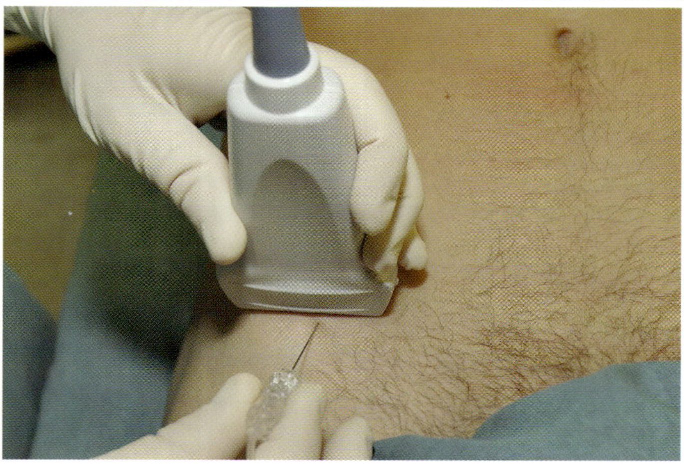

Further reading

Hurdle M, Weingarten T, Crisostomo R, Psimos C, and Smith J. Ultrasound-guided blockade of the lateral femoral cutaneous nerve: technical description and review of 10 cases. *Archives of Physical Medicine and Rehabilitation* 2007; **88**: 1362–1364.

10.7 Obturator nerve block

10.7.1 Anatomy

The obturator nerve commonly arises from the ventral divisions of L2–4. It emerges through the upper and lateral part of the obturator foramen, down to the medial side of the thigh (together with the obturator artery in the obturator canal), and divides into an anterior (between the adductor longus and adductor brevis muscles) and a posterior branch (between the adductor brevis and adductor magnus muscles).

10.7.1 *Anatomical variations*

The obturator nerve may arise from the ventral rami L1–4 (prefixed plexus) or L2–5 (postfixed plexus). Both branches of the nerve have been found to pass posterior to the adductor brevis muscle. An accessory obturator nerve may be encountered arising from L3–4 most commonly (also L2–4, L2–3, or L3). It usually runs together with the obturator nerve, but descends along the psoas major muscle to cross the anterior brim of the pelvis. The accessory obturator nerve passes beneath the pectineus muscle to terminate in three branches. These branches supply the adductor muscles and the hip joint in a variable manner.

10.7.2 Ultrasound guidance technique

The probe should be carefully moved from its position above the greater femoral vessels in a medial direction until the pectineus, long adductor, and short adductor muscles are visualized. The anterior branch of the obturator nerve is located inside this typical 'muscular triangle' (Figure 10.11). Visualization of this nerve can sometimes be improved by injection of the local anaesthetic solution. The posterior branch is located between the adductor brevis and magnus muscles.

10.7.3 Practical block technique

Both nerves should be approached by means of the IP technique and the needle inserted laterally from the probe. Advancement of the needle between the pectineus and long adductor muscle (Figures 10.12 and 10.13) avoids unnecessary tissue damage.

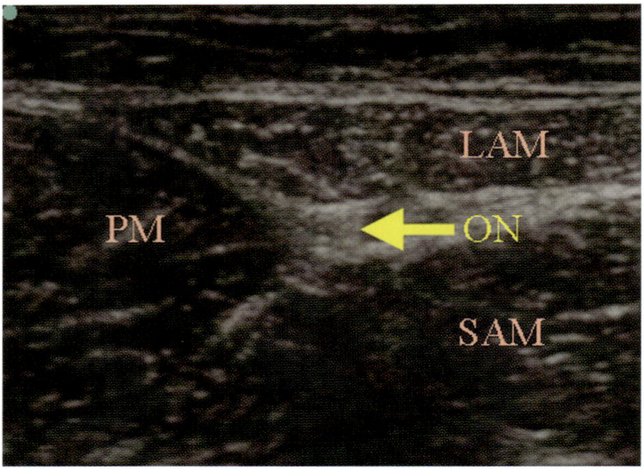

Figure 10.11 Ultrasonographic appearance of the anterior branch of the obturator nerve (ON) between the pectineus (PM), long adductor (LAM), and short adductor (SAM) muscles at the medial side of the thigh (left side = lateral).

Figure 10.12 Obturator nerve blockade. Position of the needle relative to the probe (in-plane technique)

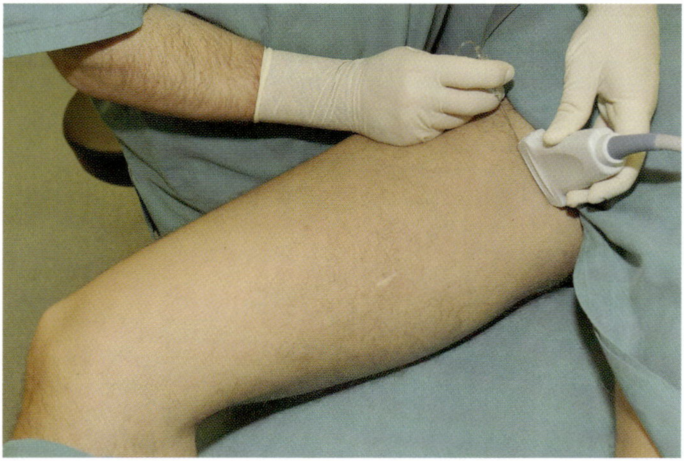

Figure 10.13 In-plane position of the needle between the pectineus and long adductor muscles for blockade of the obturator nerve (ON). The white arrow indicates the local anaesthetic solution (left side = lateral)

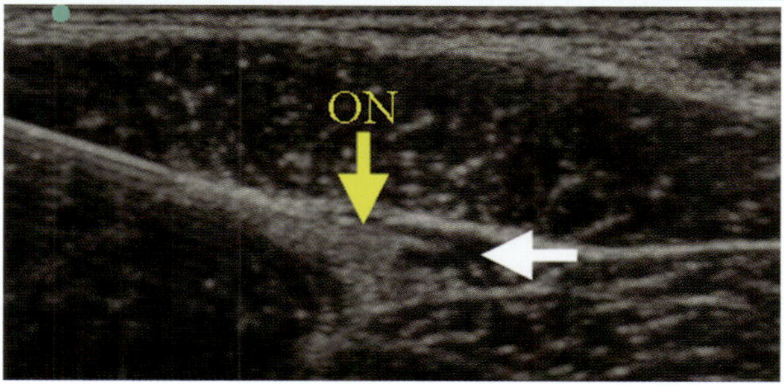

Essentials

Block characteristic	Intermediate technique
Patient position	Supine, outside rotated leg
Ultrasound equipment	Linear probe
Specific ultrasound setting	High frequency
Important anatomical structures	Pectineus, long and short adductor muscles
Ultrasound appearance of neuronal structures	Hyperechoic, round
Expected Vienna score	2–3
Needle equipment	50 or 70 mm, Facette tip
Technique	IP
Estimated local anaesthetic volume	3–4 mL each

Further reading

Soong J, Schaffhalter-Zoppoth I, and Gray A. Sonographic imaging of the obturator nerve for regional block. *Regional Anaesthesia and Pain Medicine* 2007; **32**: 146–151.

10.8 Sciatic nerve blocks

Various approaches to the sciatic nerve are possible using ultrasound-guided techniques. In the following sections we discuss five approaches: transgluteal, anterior, subgluteal, midfemoral, and popliteal. These range from proximal to distal along the sciatic nerve, until it divides into the common peroneal and tibial nerves. Despite the fact that the sciatic nerve is the largest nerve in the human body, ultrasound visualization is sometimes difficult. This might be due to the lack of easy identifiable landmarks such as large vessels and remarkable anisotropic behaviour. Careful probe adjustment and profound anatomical knowledge are necessary for reliable identification of the sciatic nerve at all levels.

10.8.1 Transgluteal approach

10.8.1.1 *Anatomy*

The sciatic nerve usually arises from the ventral rami L4–S3. Once the sciatic nerve passes out of the pelvis through the infrapiriformic foramen, it is located between the piriformis, greater gluteus, gemelli, and quadratus femoris muscles, and is accompanied medially by the posterior femoral cutaneous nerve. Since several branches supply the hip joint, this approach should be used as part of a regional anaesthesia concept for hip surgery.

10.8.1.2 *Anatomical variations*

In most cases the sciatic nerve passes beneath the piriformis muscle. In minor proportions the nerve may pierce the latter (most frequently only the peroneal part) or pass above the piriformis muscle. The level of division into common peroneal and tibial nerves may be encountered at any level between its origin the lower thigh.

10.8.1.3 *Ultrasound guidance technique*

The deep location of the sciatic nerve from a transgluteal approach requires that a sector probe be used. Optimally, the patient should be positioned laterally, with a slightly flexed hip and knee. The probe should be placed in a connecting line between the coccygeus and the greater trochanter. The sciatic nerves can be expected to lie at a depth of 5–8 cm and to be visible as as hyperechoic, flat to round structures (Figure 10.14). Due to the need for low to middle frequencies for this approach, the internal structure of the nerve cannot be visualized. With the probe positioned as described above, the cutaneous femoris posterior nerve is constantly medial to the sciatic nerve and direct visualization may be difficult due to the small diameter of the nerve.

Figure 10.14 Ultrasonographic appearance of the sciatic nerve (SN) between the greater trochanter (GT) and the sciatic tuber (ST) at the transgluteal level (left side = lateral). GGM: greater gluteus muscle

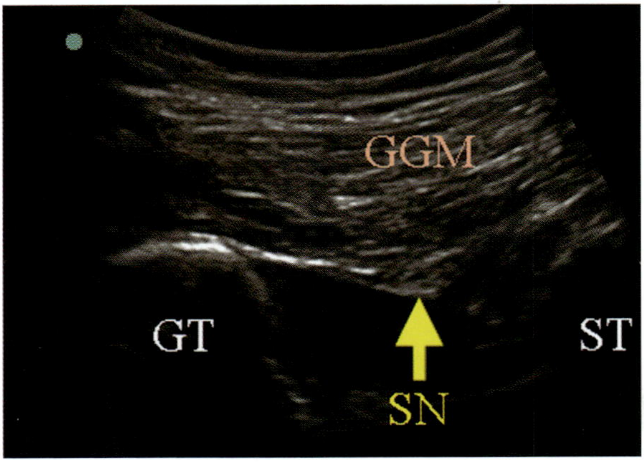

10.8.1.4 *Practical block technique*

Once the sciatic nerve is adequately visualized, the block should be performed using an OOP technique (Figure 10.15). At least two needle positions are necessary for a successful blockade: one lateral and one medial to the nerve. Administering a larger volume of local anaesthetic at the medial side also blocks the cutaneous femoris posterior nerve. Due to the depth of the block, however, direct visualization of the tip of the needle may be difficult and requires good hand–eye coordination skills. Careful observation of the additional signs of the position of the needle (e.g., movement of the tissues, shadow behind the tip of the needle) is mandatory. Nevertheless, observation of the spread of local anaesthetic is easily achieved. It is important to note that the block takes longer to work than others for proximal sciatic nerve blockade.

Essentials

Block characteristic	Intermediate technique
Patient position	Lateral, hip and knee slightly flexed
Ultrasound equipment	Sector probe
Specific ultrasound setting	Middle to low frequency
Important anatomical structures	Greater gluteus, gemelli, and quadratus femoris muscles
Ultrasound appearance of neuronal structures	Hyperechoic, round to oval
Expected Vienna score	3
Needle equipment	80–120 mm, Facette tip
Technique	IP
Estimated local anaesthetic volume	12–16 mL

Figure 10.15 Transgluteal sciatic nerve blockade. Position of the needle relative to the probe (out-of-plane technique)

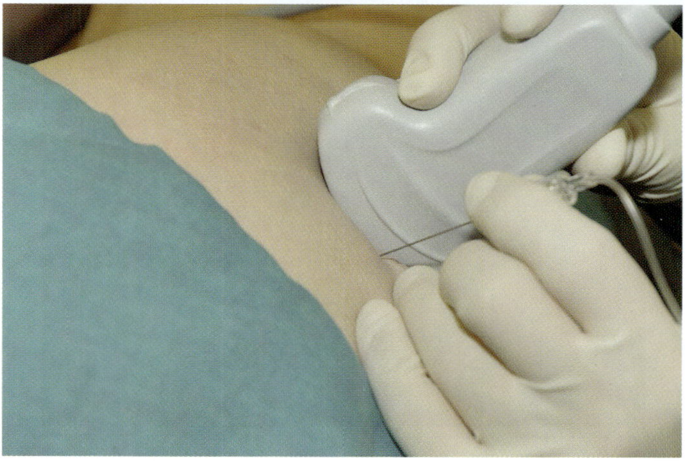

10.8.2 Anterior approach

10.8.2.1 *Anatomy*

See other proximal approaches to the sciatic nerve.

10.8.2.2 *Ultrasound guidance technique*

Using the anterior technique, the sciatic nerve can be visualized between the minor trochanter and the sciatic tuber. Although the sciatic nerve is in its deepest position using the anterior approach, the technique is relatively comfortable for the patient from the positioning point of view (supine). Once the minor trochanter and sciatic tuber are visualized, the nerve is situated between these bony structures and below the rectus femoris and greater adductor muscles (Figure 10.16). A low-frequency sector probe should be used, and the nerve should appear as a hyperechoic, round to oval structure.

10.8.2.3 *Practical block technique*

Once the nerve is visualized between the minor trochanter and sciatic tuber, the block should be performed between the rectus femoris and sartorius muscles using the IP technique with the needle positioned in an absolute perpendicular direction from medial (Figure 10.17). The length of the needle depends on the initial measurement of the depth of the nerve; 100–120-mm needles are usually adequate. The needle should be placed both medial and lateral to the nerve. Careful aspiration is necessary prior to the administration of local anaesthetic as small vessels are difficult to visualize at the depth of the sciatic nerve.

Figure 10.16 Ultrasonographic appearance of the sciatic nerve (SN) medial to and below the femur by realizing the anterior approach (left side = lateral). GAM: greater adductor muscle

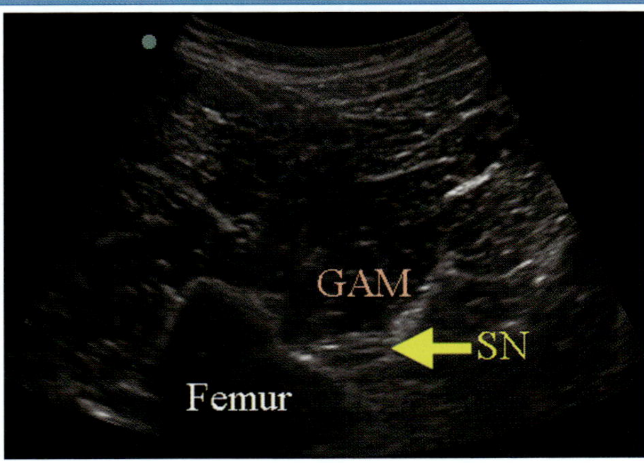

Figure 10.17 Anterior approach to the sciatic nerve. Position of the needle relative to the probe (in-plane technique)

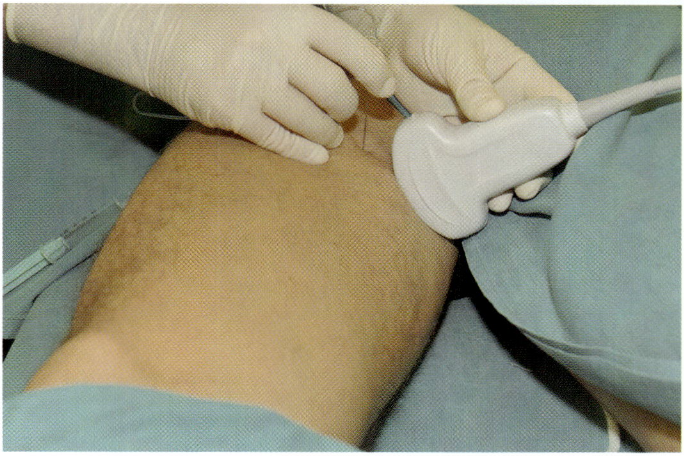

Essentials

Block characteristic	Intermediate technique
Patient position	Supine, slightly lateral rotated lower extremity
Ultrasound equipment	Sector probe
Specific ultrasound setting	Low frequency
Important anatomical structures	Minor trochanter, sciatic tuber; rectus femoris, sartorius, and greater adductor muscles
Ultrasound appearance of neuronal structures	Hyperechoic, flat to oval
Expected Vienna score	3–4
Needle equipment	100–120 mm, Facette tip
Technique	IP
Estimated local anaesthetic volume	15 mL

10.8.3 Subgluteal approach

10.8.3.1 *Anatomy*

In the subgluteal region the sciatic nerve is situated between the greater trochanter and the sciatic tuberosity, embedded between the quadriceps femoris and greater gluteus muscles. In the same layer, the posterior femoral cutaneous nerve is found medial to the sciatic nerve.

10.8.3.2 *Ultrasound guidance technique*

Ultrasound-guided blockade is an attractive option for blocking the sciatic nerve in the subgluteal fold as here it lies in a superficial position. A high-frequency, 38-mm linear probe should be used for this approach. On visualization, the nerve should appear as a hyperechoic, flat to oval structure below the greater gluteus muscle. The cutaneous femoral posterior nerve appears medial to the sciatic nerve as hyperechoic round structure (Figure 10.18).

10.8.3.3 ***Practical block technique***

We have found that three different patient positions are possible for the subgluteal approach: (1) Supine with a 90° flexed hip, (2) lateral position with a 45° flexed hip, or (3) prone. An OOP technique should be used in all cases (Figures 10.19). Once the tip of the needle is placed lateral to the nerve and some of the local anaesthetic administered, it is necessary to redirect the tip of the needle to the medial side of the nerve in order to achieve an adequate spread of local anaesthetic. In some cases, the sciatic nerve is adherent to the quadratus lumborum muscle and a complete circumferential spread cannot be achieved (which is one explanation for long sensory and motor onset times). A slight medial redirection of the needle tip should be sufficient for additional blockade of the cutaneus femoral posterior nerve.

Figure 10.18 Ultrasonographic appearance of the sciatic (SN) and cutaneous femoral posterior (CFPN) nerves at the subgluteal level (left side = lateral). GGM: greater gluteus muscle

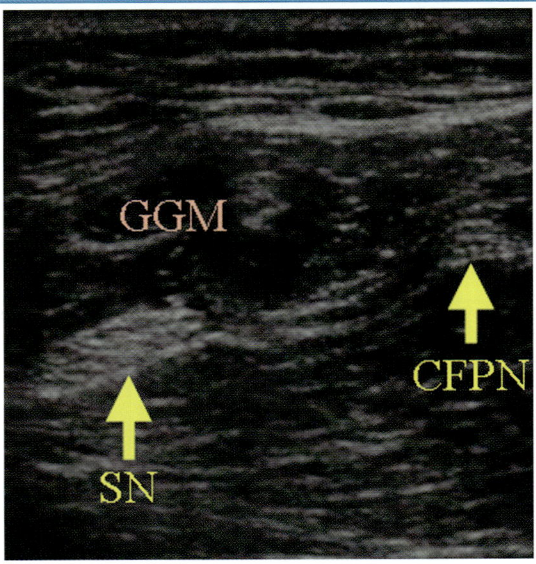

Figure 10.19 Subgluteal sciatic nerve blockade. Position of the needle relative to the probe (out-of-plane technique)

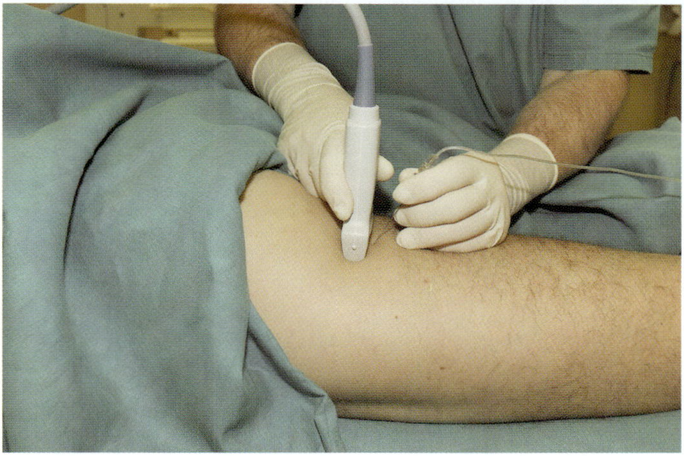

Essentials

Block characteristic	Intermediate technique
Patient position	Supine (90° flexed hip and knee), lateral (with 45° flexed hip), or prone
Ultrasound equipment	Linear probe, 38 mm
Specific ultrasound setting	High–medium frequency
Important anatomical structures	Greater gluteus muscle
Ultrasound appearance of neuronal structures	Hyperechoic, flat
Expected Vienna score	2
Needle equipment	50 mm, Facette tip
Technique	OOP
Estimated local anaesthetic volume	15 mL

10.8.4 Midfemoral approach

10.8.4.1 *Anatomy*

In the midfemoral region, the sciatic nerve lies underneath the long head of the biceps muscle. More distal, the nerve is positioned between the long head of the biceps (lateral side of the nerve) and the semitendinosus muscles (medial side of the nerve).

10.8.4.2 *Ultrasound guidance technique*

The best visibility of the sciatic nerve in the midfemoral region of the thigh can be achieved between the long head of the biceps and the semitendinosus muscles. A high-frequency, 38-mm linear probe should be used. Careful probe adjustments should provide optimal visibility of the nerve as a hyperechoic, round to oval structure (Figure 10.20).

Figure 10.20 Ultrasonographic appearance of the sciatic nerve (SN) at the midfemoral level (left side = lateral). LHBM: long head of the biceps muscle; STM: semitendinosus muscle

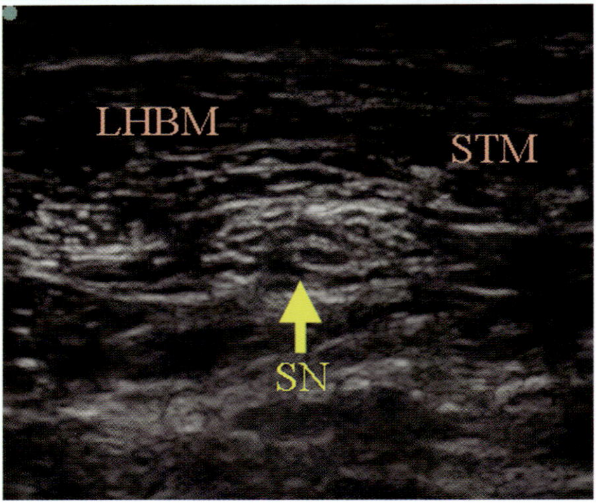

10.8.4.3 ***Practical block technique***

Lateral position of the patient with slightly flexed hip and knee is a comfortable and practical patient position for that approach to the sciatic nerve. Prone position is also an option. After visualization of the nerve between the long head of the biceps and semitendinosus muscles, the needle should be carefully advanced between those two muscles using the OOP technique (Figure 10.21). As described for the more proximal approaches to the sciatic nerve, both medial and lateral needle tip positioning is mandatory for a circumferential spread of local anaesthetic.

Essentials

Block characteristic	Intermediate technique
Patient position	Lateral, slightly flexed hip and knee; prone
Ultrasound equipment	Linear probe, 38 mm
Specific ultrasound setting	High frequency
Important anatomical structures	Long head biceps and semitendinosus muscles
Ultrasound appearance of neuronal structures	Hyperechoic, round to oval
Expected Vienna score	2
Needle equipment	50–70 mm, Facette tip
Technique	OOP
Estimated local anaesthetic volume	12–15 mL

Figure 10.21 Midfemoral approach to the sciatic nerve. Position of the needle relative to the probe (out-of-plane technique)

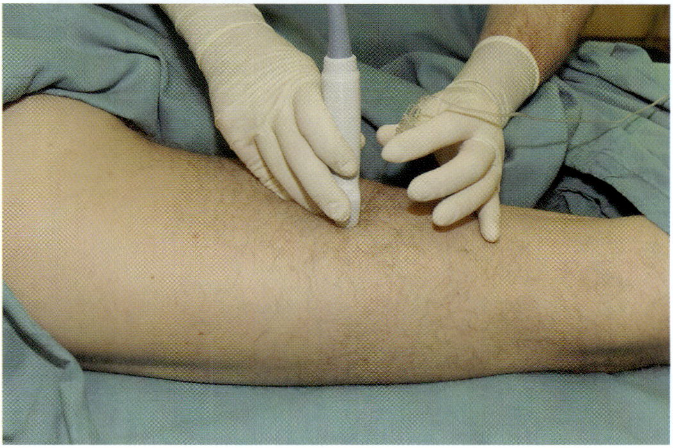

10.8.5 Popliteal approach

10.8.5.1 *Anatomy*

In the popliteal area, the sciatic nerve is usually divided into its tibial and common peroneal branches. The main sciatic nerve is situated between the biceps femoris (lateral side) and semimembranosus (medial side) muscles lateral to the popliteal vessels. The common peroneal nerve runs laterally below the lateral head of the gastrocnemius muscle, and the tibial nerve runs between the medial and lateral head of the gastrocnemius muscle to give off the sural nerve.

10.8.5.2 *Ultrasound guidance technique*

First, a high-frequency linear probe should be used to detect the sciatic nerve from the popliteal fossa as a hyperechoic round structure. Next, the nerve should be tracked in a distal direction until the division into its tibial and common peroneus branches can be observed (Figure 10.22). Both the tibial and common peroneus nerves are less echogenic in comparison with the main sciatic nerve.

10.8.5.3 *Practical block technique*

With the patient in a supine position, the hip and knee flexed, the probe should be placed from a dorsal position to detect the main sciatic nerve. The block should be performed proximal to the division, except in cases where a selective blockade of the tibial or common peroneus nerves is required. Once the needle is introduced below the biceps muscle, the tip should be placed using the IP technique above and below the nerve to achieve a circumferential spread of local anaesthetic (Figures 10.23 and 10.24). The techniques to block the tibial and common peroneus nerves are identical.

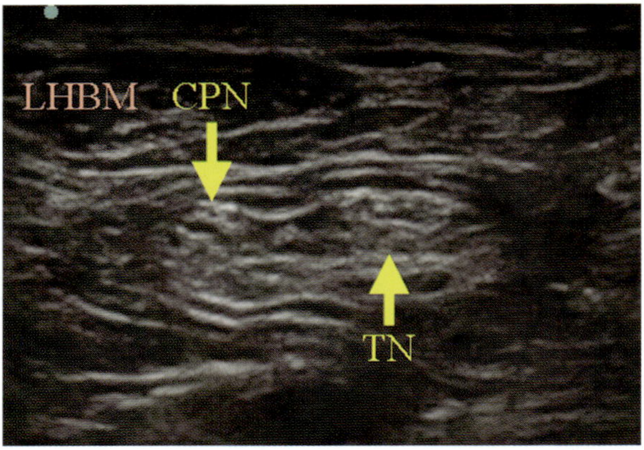

Figure 10.22 Ultrasonographic appearance of the common peroneus (CPN) and tibial (TN) tibial nerves slightly distal the sciatic nerve division (left side = lateral). LHBM: long head of the biceps femoral muscle.

Figure 10.23 Popliteal approach to the sciatic nerve. Position of the needle relative to the probe (in-plane technique)

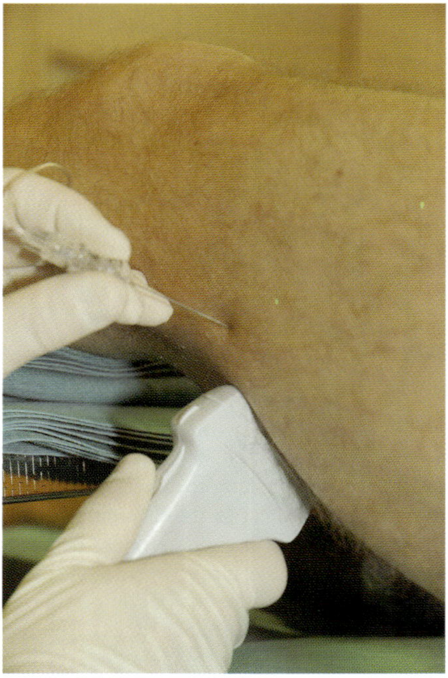

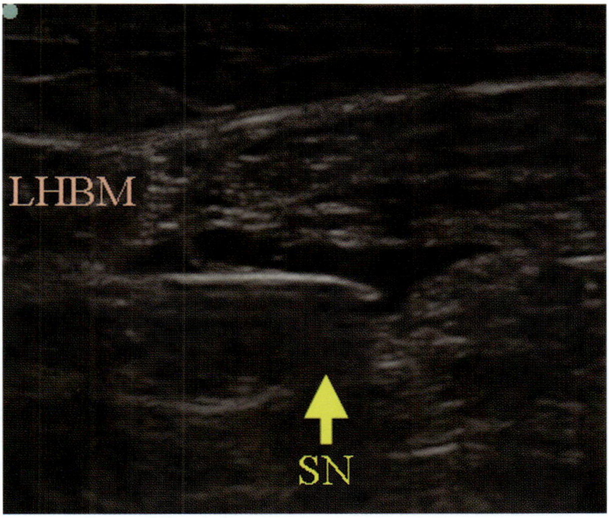

Figure 10.24 In-plane needle guidance technique for the sciatic nerve (SN) blockade at the popliteal level slightly proximal to the division. Large parts of the sciatic nerve are hidden by the body of the needle (left side = lateral). LHBM: long head of the biceps femoral muscle.

Essentials

Block characteristic	Intermediate technique
Patient position	Supine, hip and knee flexed, pillow under the ankle
Ultrasound equipment	Linear probe, 38 mm
Specific ultrasound setting	High frequency
Important anatomical structures	Biceps and semimembranosus muscles, popliteal vessels
Ultrasound appearance of neuronal structures	Main sciatic nerve: hyperechoic, round Tibial and common peroneus nerves: less hyper-echoic in comparison to sciatic nerve, round
Expected Vienna score	Main sciatic nerve: 2 Tibial and common peroneus nerves: 3
Needle equipment	50–70 mm, Facette tip
Technique	IP
Estimated local anaesthetic volume	15 mL

Further reading

Oberndorfer U, Marhofer P, Bösenberg A *et al.* Ultrasonographic guidance for sciatic and femoral nerve blocks in children. *British Journal of Anaesthesia* 2007; **98**: 797–801.

Chan V, Nova H, Abbas S, McCartney C, Perlas A, and Xu D. Ultrasound examination and localization of the sciatic nerve: a volunteer study. *Anesthesiology* 2006; **104**: 309–314.

10.9 Ankle blocks

Despite the popularity of ankle nerve blocks for foot surgery, the descriptions of these blocks in the literature are based purely on superficial anatomical landmarks. None of them are described in sufficient scientific manner. As compensation for these weak descriptions, relatively large volumes of local anaesthetics are recommended for ankle block techniques, with subsequent pain during injection due to the fact that tense tendons and muscles are in close proximity to the nerves.

Most types of foot surgery usually require the blockade of the tibial nerve, as well as the profound and superficial branches of the peroneus nerve.

10.9.1 Tibial nerve

10.9.1.2 *Anatomy*

The tibial nerve passes posterior to the medial malleolus, closely adjacent to the posterior tibial artery and vein. The tendons of the tibialis posterior and flexor digitorum longus muscles are situated anterior to the nerve. The tendon of the flexor hallucis longus muscle lies posterior to the tibial nerve.

10.9.1.3 *Anatomical variations*

Variations in the arrangement of the tibial nerve around the vessels are possible.

10.9.1.4 *Ultrasound guidance technique*

A high-frequency, 25-mm linear probe should be used, with optimal positioning slightly proximal to the medial malleolus. The posterior tibial artery is a major landmark and the tibial nerve can be visualized as a hyperechoic round structure close to the artery (Figure 10.25).

10.9.1.5 *Practical block technique*

After optimal visualization of the tibial nerve with the probe positioned slightly proximal to the medial malleolus, the block should be performed using the OOP technique (Figure 10.26) Only a small volume (1–2 mL) of local anaesthetic is required. Prior to the block, careful aspiration is mandatory since several veins are located around the nerve.

Essentials

Block characteristic	Basic technique
Patient position	Supine, outside rotated lower leg
Ultrasound equipment	Linear probe, 25 mm
Specific ultrasound setting	High frequency
Important anatomical structures	Posterior tibial artery
Ultrasound appearance of neuronal structures	Hyperechoic, round
Expected Vienna score	2
Needle equipment	30–50 mm, Facette tip
Technique	OOP
Estimated local anaesthetic volume	1–2 mL

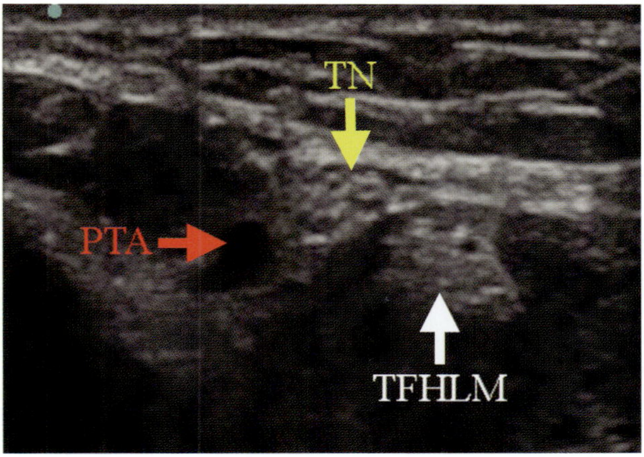

Figure 10.25 Ultrasonographic appearance of the tibial nerve (TN) slightly cranial the medial malleolus (left side = anterior). PTA: posterior tibial artery; TFHLM: tendon of the flexor hallucis longus muscle.

Figure 10.26 Tibial nerve blockade. Position of the needle relative to the probe (out-of-plane technique).

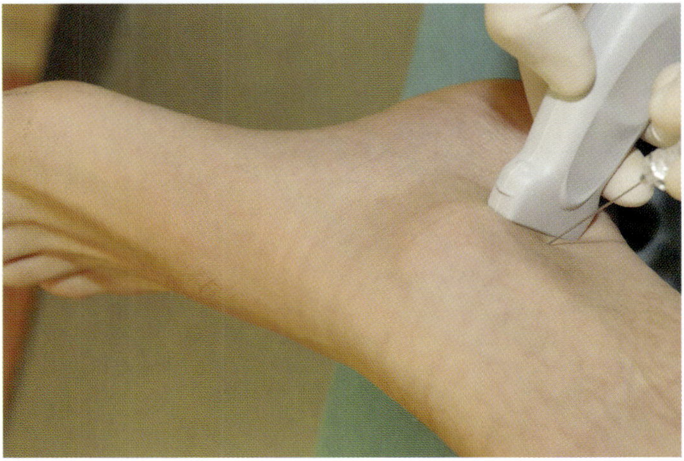

10.9.2 Profound branch of the peroneus nerve

10.9.2.1 *Anatomy*

The profound branch of the peroneal nerve takes its course laterally to the anterior tibial artery in a distal direction.

10.9.2.2 *Anatomical variations*

Absence of this branch and substitute innervation by saphenous and sural nerves have been described.

10.9.2.3 *Ultrasound guidance technique*

A high-frequency, 25-mm linear probe should be placed at the medial lateral side of the distal lower leg. The nerve can be detected between the extensor hallucis longus and extensor digitorum longus muscles as a hyperechoic round structure (Figure 10.27).

10.9.2.4 *Practical block technique*

The block should be performed using the OOP technique with the needle directed between the extensor hallucis longus and extensor digitorum longus muscles (Figure 10.28). Care should be taken to avoid puncture of the anterior tibial artery.

Essentials

Block characteristic	Basic technique
Patient position	Supine, neural leg position
Ultrasound equipment	Linear probe, 25 mm
Specific ultrasound setting	High frequencies
Important anatomical structures	Anterior tibial artery
Ultrasound appearance of neuronal structures	Hyperechoic, round
Expected Vienna score	2
Needle equipment	50 mm, Facette tip
Technique	OOP
Estimated local anaesthetic volume	1–2 mL

10.9.3 Superficial branch of the peroneus nerve

10.9.3.1 *Anatomy*

The superficial branch of the peroneus nerve runs at the mid-level of the lower leg, between the short and long fibular muscles at the lateral side. Above the lateral malleolus, the nerve is situated very superficially above the deep fascia which forms the superior extensor retinaculum.

10.9.3.2 *Anatomical variations*

Absence of this nerve and substitute innervation by the saphenous and sural nerves have been described.

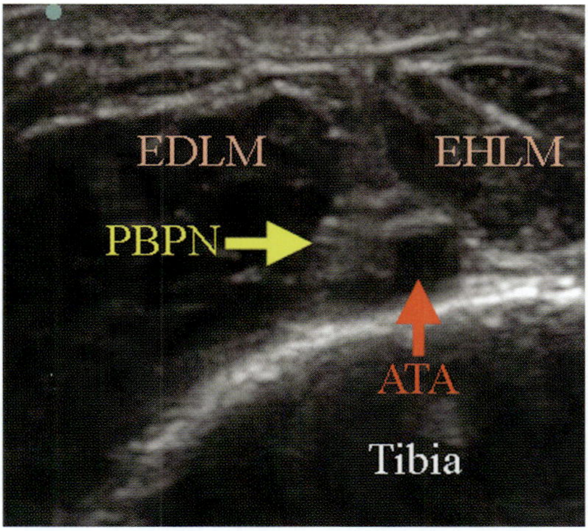

Figure 10.27 Ultrasonographic appearance of the profound branch of the peroneus nerve (PBPN) close to the anterior tibial artery (ATA) between the extensor tibialis (left side = lateral). EDLM: extensor digitorum longus muscle; EHLM: extensor hallucis longus muscle).

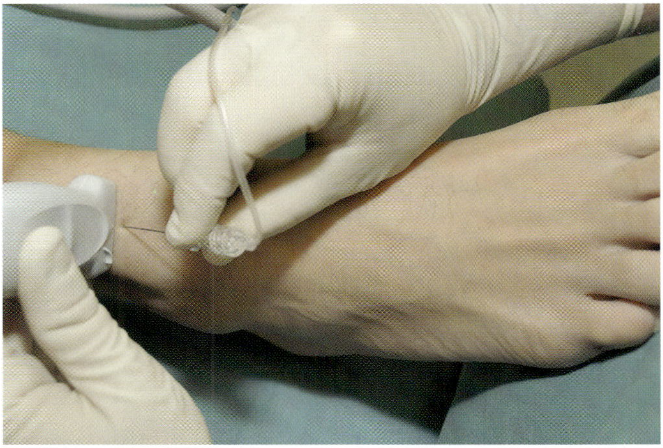

Figure 10.28 Blockade of the profound branch of the tibial nerve. Position of the needle relative to the probe (out-of-plane technique)

10.9.3.3 *Ultrasound guidance technique*

Placing a high-frequency, 25-mm linear probe cranial and anterior to the lateral malleolus, the peroneus nerve appears as a small hyperechoic round structure (Figure 10.29). Ultrasonographic identification of the nerve may be difficult due to a lack of clearly demarcated landmarks.

10.9.3.4 ***Practical block technique***

Once the nerve is identified, an OOP technique should be employed to block the nerve (Figure 10.30). If safe identification of the nerve proves difficult, a more proximal approach should be used.

Figure 10.29 Ultrasonographic appearance of the superficial branch of the peroneus nerve (SBPN) where it pierces the fascia (left side = lateral)

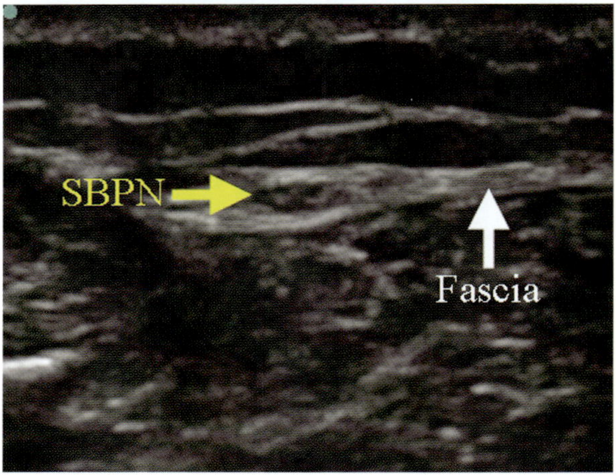

Figure 10.30 Blockade of the superficial branch of the tibial nerve. Position of the needle relative to the probe (out-of-plane technique)

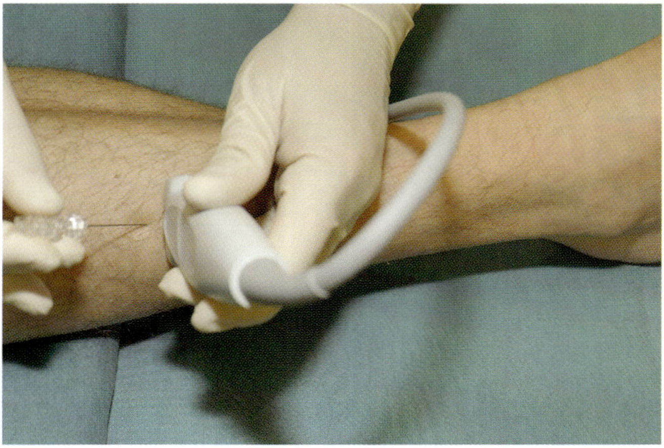

Essentials

Block characteristic	Basic technique
Patient position	Supine, neutral leg position
Ultrasound equipment	Linear probe, 25 mm
Specific ultrasound setting	High frequency
Important anatomical structures	–
Ultrasound appearance of neuronal structures	Hyperechoic, round
Expected Vienna score	2–3
Needle equipment	OOP
Technique	50 mm, Facette tip
Estimated local anaesthetic volume	1–2 mL

Chapter 11

Truncal blocks

Truncal blocks are well established regional anaesthetic techniques in the abdominal region, providing pain relief by blocking the sensory end branches of the ventral rami Th7–12 and L1–2. Historically, blind techniques relying on tactile sensation ('scratching sensations' or 'palpable gives') to identify the correct needle position have been the standard method for these nerve blocks. These simple but often forgotten blocks can be divided into three techniques:

- *Intercostal nerve blocks* provide analgesia for thoracic and upper abdominal surgery. Blockade of two dermatomes above and two below the level of surgery is required for an adequate analgesia.
- *Ilioinguinal/iliohypogastric* nerve blocks are common analgesic techniques for providing adequate pain relief during inguinal surgery.
- *Rectus sheath blocks* provide effective pain relief for umbilical or other midline surgical approaches. This regional anaesthetic technique was first described by Schleich in 1899 to provide relaxation of the anterior abdominal wall by blocking the terminal branches of intercostal nerves 9–11 within the rectus sheath.

11.1 Intercostal blocks

11.1.1 Anatomy

The intercostal nerves supply the skin and the muscles of the chest and the abdominal wall. They can be visualized at the dorsum of the thorax, between the pleura and the posterior intercostal membrane. After a short distance they pierce the posterior intercostal membrane and run between the two planes of intercostal muscles. After approximately two-thirds of their course, the intercostal nerves enter and run within the fibres of the intercostales interni muscles. As they near the costal cartilages, the nerves reach the inner surface of the intercostales interni muscles and subsequently run below the pleura. Finally, the intercostal nerves pass inferior to the respective rib, together with the intercostal vessels.

11.1.1.1 *Anatomical variations*

Thoracic spinal roots, as well as ventral rami, may be absent.

11.1.2 Ultrasound guidance technique

Due to the sonic shadow of the rib it is not possible to visualize intercostal nerves. It is therefore essential to define the external and internal intercostal muscles, and the pleura (Figure 11.1). Administration of 1.5-mL local anaesthetic

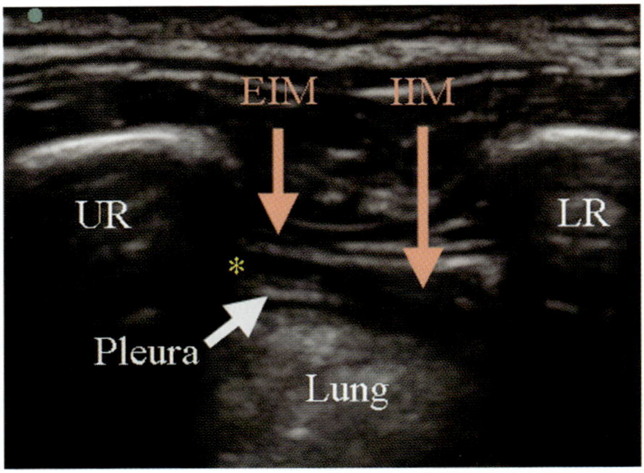

Figure 11.1 Ultrasonographic identification of external (EIM) and internal intercostal (IIM) muscles and pleura (left side = cranial). UR: upper rib; LR: lower rib; asterisks indicate the injection point of local anaesthetic.

is usually sufficient when administered within the internal intercostal muscle to fill up the entire intercostal space. With this amount of local anaesthetic, it is also possible to block the collateral branch on the upper border of the caudal rib.

11.1.3 Practical block technique

After exact identification of the ribs, the external and internal intercostal muscles, and the pleura in the posterior axillary line, the needle is inserted by the OOP technique with the transducer positioned transverse to the ribs (Figure 11.2). The needle should be inserted very carefully into the external intercostal muscle. The correct position of the tip of the needle within the external intercostal muscle can be verified by injecting very small amounts (0.2 mL) of local anaesthetic. Once verified, the needle should be advanced carefully within the internal intercostal muscle and, upon correct positioning, 1.5 mL of local anaesthetic is injected.

Essentials

Block characteristic	Basic technique
Patient position	Supine, thorax slightly lateral rotated
Ultrasound equipment	Linear probe, 38 mm
Specific ultrasound setting	High frequencies
Important anatomical structures	External and internal intercostal muscles, pleura
Ultrasound appearance of neuronal structures	–
Expected Vienna score	–
Needle equipment	50 mm, Facette tip
Technique	OOP
Estimated local anaesthetic volume	1.5 mL

Figure 11.2 Position of the needle relative to the probe for an intercostal block (out-of-plane technique)

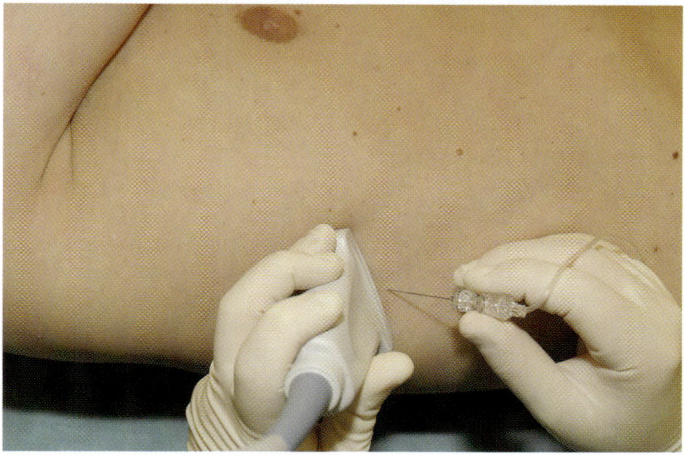

11.2 Ilioinguinal/iliohypogastric nerve blocks

11.2.1 Anatomy

The iliohypogastric nerves is formed by the ventral ramus L1 and a branch of T12. It emerges from the lateral border of the psoas major muscle, passes across the ventral surface of the quadratus lumborum, and descends to the iliac crest. As it nears the anterior superior iliac spine, the nerve pierces the transverse abdominal muscle to take its course beneath the internal oblique and transverse abdominal muscles. The ilioinguinal nerve, which is formed by the ventral rami L1–2 follows a similar course.

11.2.1.1 *Anatomical variations*

Both nerves occasionally arise as a common trunk, only to become separated between the transverse and internal oblique muscles. The iliohypogastric nerve sometimes arises from the subcostal nerve, it may also receive a branch from the 11th thoracic nerve. In some cases, the ilioinguinal nerve may terminate near the iliac crest to join the iliohypogastric nerve, whereupon branches of the iliohypogastric nerve replace the absent fibres. A lateral cutaneous or iliac branch may arise to supply the skin in the region of the anterior superior iliac spine. It may also replace the genital branch of the genitofemoral nerve or the lateral femoral cutaneous nerve. In rare cases, the ilioinguinal nerve is absent altogether.

11.2.2 Ultrasound guidance technique

In adults, the ilioinguinal and iliohypogastric nerves are best visible a few centimetres cranial and lateral to the anterior superior iliac spine. Here, the nerves can usually be found situated between the internal oblique abdominal muscle and the transverse abdominal muscle. Figure 11.3 shows a typical ultrasound picture of this region. The position of the ultrasound probe is transverse in relation to the nerves.

11.2.3 Practical block technique

After identification of the ilioinguinal and iliohypogastric nerves, the block is performed using the OOP technique. In general, it is possible to place the tip of the needle between the ilioinguinal and iliohypogastric nerves and inject about 10 mL (0.1 mL/kg) of local anaesthetic to achieve an adequate distribution. In patients with chronic pain, it is possible to distinguish whether a pain syndrome is caused by either the iliohypogastric or ilioinguinal nerve by blocking each nerve with 1 mL of local anaesthetic. For this purpose, diffusion of local anaesthetic along a fascial plane should be avoided. Figures 11.4 and 11.5 illustrate the OOP needle guidance technique and a typical ultrasound picture of the puncture site after injection. The needle is placed in between both nerves.

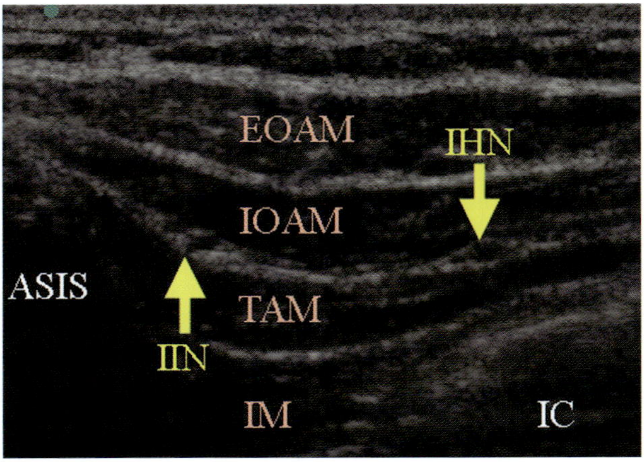

Figure 11.3 Ultrasonographic illustration of the lateral abdominal wall at the level of the anterior superior iliac spine (left side = lateral). ASIS: anterior superior iliac spine; EOAM: external oblique abdominal muscle; IC: intraperitoneal cavum; IHN: iliohypogastric nerve; IIN: ilioinguinal nerve; IM: iliac muscle; IOAM: internal oblique abdominal muscle; TAM: transverse abdominal muscle.

Figure 11.4 Ilioinguinal/iliohypogastric nerve block. Position of the needle relative to the probe (out-of-plane technique)

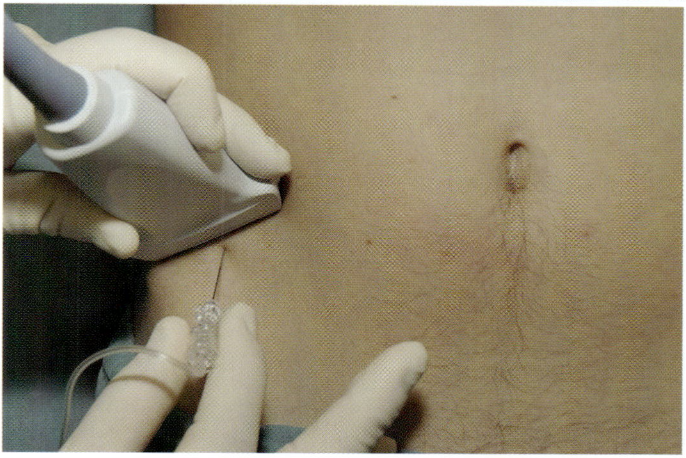

Figure 11.5 Ilioinguinal/iliohypogastric (IIN/IHN) nerve block with 10 mL local anaesthetic (indicated by the white arrows) (left side = lateral)

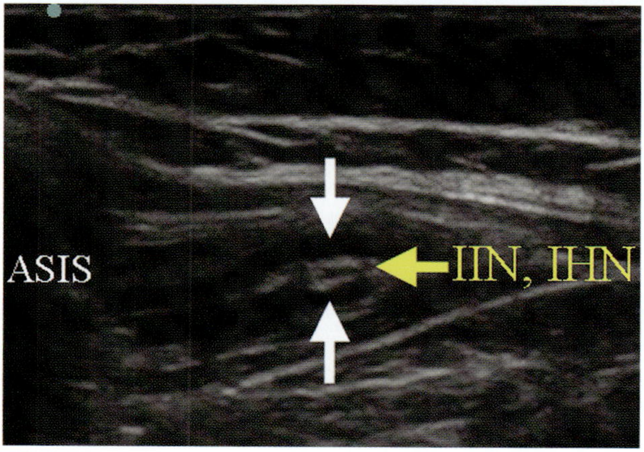

Essentials

Block characteristic	Basic technique
Patient position	Supine
Ultrasound equipment	Linear probe, 38 mm
Specific ultrasound setting	High frequency
Important anatomical structures	External oblique, internal oblique, and transverse abdominal muscles
Ultrasound appearance of neuronal structures	Round and oval hyperechoic nerves
Expected Vienna score	1–2
Needle equipment	50 mm, Facette tip
Technique	OOP
Estimated local anaesthetic volume	5–10 mL (0.1 mL/kg)

Further reading

Eichenberger U, Greher M, Kirchmair L, Curatolo M, and Moriggl B. Ultrasound-guided blocks of the ilioinguinal and iliohypogastric nerve: accuracy of a selective new technique confirmed by anatomical dissection. *British Journal of Anaesthesia* 2006; **97**: 238–243.

Willschke H, Marhofer P, Bösenberg A *et al.* Ultrasonography for ilioinguinal/iliohypogastric nerve blocks in children. *British Journal of Anaesthesia* 2005; **95**: 226–230.

11.3 Rectus sheath block

11.3.1 Anatomy

The central abdominal wall consists of rectus abdominal muscle, which is embedded in the anterior and posterior rectus sheath. These fascial sheaths are formed by the aponeuroses of the transverse, internal oblique, and external oblique abdominal muscles. There are three tendinous intersections within the rectus abdominis muscle, one at the level of the xiphoid, one at the umbilicus, and one in between. The intercostal nerves 9–11 pass behind the costal cartilage and between the internal oblique and the transverse abdominis muscle. Usually, the nerves run between the posterior rectus sheath and the posterior wall of the rectus abdominis muscle. Ultimately, they perforate the sheath with their anterior cutaneus branches supplying the skin in the midline.

11.3.1.1 *Anatomical variations*

It has been reported that parts or even the whole of the rectus abdominis muscle may be absent or doubled. Numerous variations concerning the origins and insertions of the abdominal muscles have been described, but seem to have no impact on the described technique of rectus sheath block.

11.3.2 Ultrasound guidance technique

The main difference to most other peripheral regional anaesthetic techniques is that the local anaesthetic is injected next to a fascial plane without direct visualization of nerve structures. Diffusion along this plane will transport the local anaesthetic to the terminal branches of the intercostal nerves. Using ultrasonography, it is possible to place the local anaesthetic in between the posterior rectus sheath and the rectus abdominis muscle. We recommend placing the ultrasound probe in a transverse position in relation to the rectus abdominal muscle.

11.3.3 Practical block technique

After exact identification of the rectus abdominis muscle and the posterior rectus sheath, the block is performed bilaterally at the level of the umbilicus using an OOP technique (Figures 11.6 and 11.7). Once the tip of the needle is correctly positioned between the rectus abdominis muscle and the posterior rectus sheath, a predetermined volume of 0.1 mL/kg local anaesthetic will be injected (Figure 11.8).

Figure 11.6 Ultrasonographic illustration of the posterior rectus sheath (PRS) lateral to the umbilicus (left side = lateral). RAM: rectus abdominis muscle

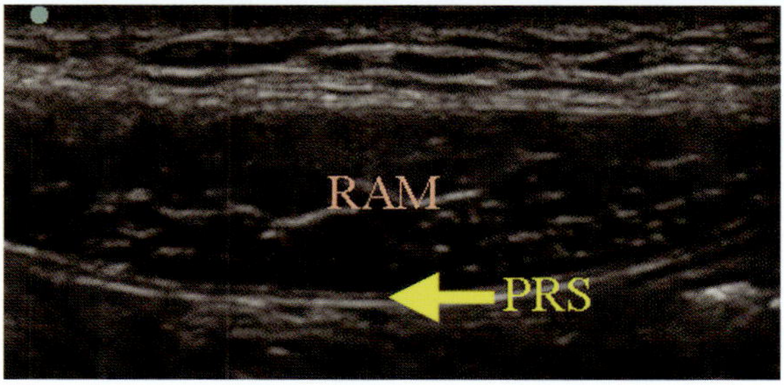

Figure 11.7 Out-of-plane needle guidance technique for the rectus sheath block

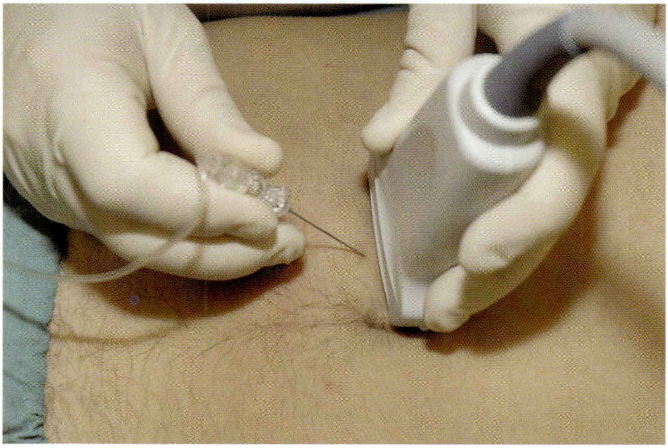

Figure 11.8 Rectus sheath block with 0.1 mL/kg local anaesthetic (indicated by the white arrow) (left side = medial). RAM: rectus abdominis muscle; U: umbilicus

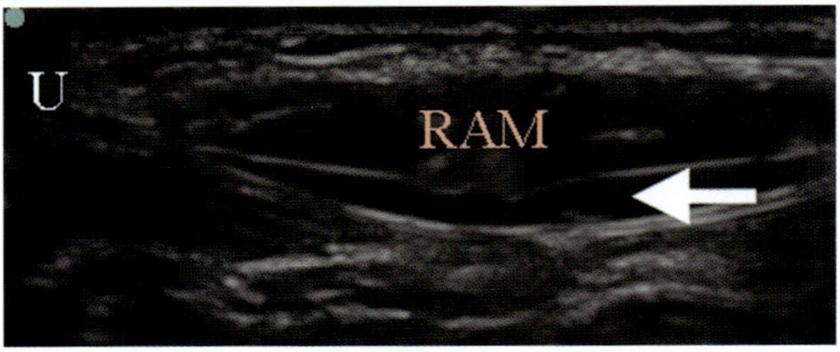

Essentials

Block characteristic	Basic technique
Patient position	Supine
Ultrasound equipment	Linear probe
Specific ultrasound setting	High frequency
Important anatomical structures	Rectus abdominis muscle, anterior and posterior rectus sheath
Ultrasound appearance of neuronal structures	–
Expected Vienna score	–
Needle equipment	50 mm, Facette tip
Technique	OOP
Estimated local anaesthetic volume	0.1 mL/kg/side

Further reading

Willschke H, Bösenberg A, Marhofer P *et al.* Ultrasonographic-guided rectus sheath block in paediatric anaesthesia: a new approach to an old technique. *British Journal of Anaesthesia* 2006; **97**: 244–249.

Chapter 12

Catheter techniques

All catheter techniques can be performed as either single or continuous techniques: the degree of visualization of the nerves is equal. During positioning, the catheter could be directly visualized in most cases (Figure 12.1). More importantly, the spread of local anaesthetic was able to be observed. We suggest the use of adhesive, transparent tape for fixation of a peripheral nerve block catheter, so that a daily ultrasonographic investigation of the spread of local anaesthetic is possible.

Using ultrasound to detect the spread of local anaesthetic enables important information to be gathered about the optimal block mechanism of specific approaches. Despite a lack of scientific studies of catheter approaches, we have been able to conduct an initial evaluation of useful techniques. Due to the fact that ultrasound-guided regional block techniques are strictly performed using multi-injections, we were able to make the following recommendations:

For continuous blockade of the upper extremity, the interscalene and supraclavicular approaches are advisable, made more attractive as they are less hampered than other approaches by the close proximity of the nerve structures in this region. Due to superficial neuronal structures, the spread of local anaesthetic relative to nerves and the catheter can be visualized.

For lower extremity blocks, femoral and midfemoral sciatic catheter techniques should be performed. Particular care should be taken with the sciatic approach due to the large diameter of the nerve. If this proves problematic, the catheter should be carefully adjusted until the local anaesthetic surrounds the nerve circumferentially.

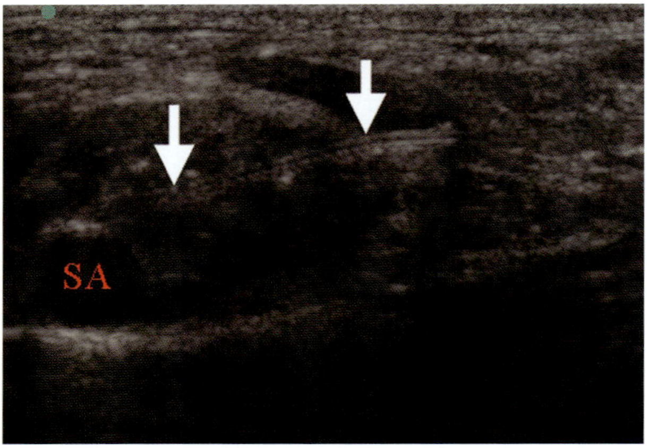

Figure 12.1 Direct ultrasonographic visualization of a catheter (indicated by the white arrows) with the tip above the subclavian artery (SA) for a continuous supraclavicular plexus blockade.

Chapter 13

Future perspectives

13.1 Education

Currently, learning tools for, education about, and certification of the use of ultrasound-guided regional anaesthesia are under discussion. The consensus is that new learning tools are required to improve teaching in this fast-growing field of anaesthesia. Most of the traditional textbooks already include chapters concerning ultrasound-guided nerve blockade, and new textbooks such as this that focus solely on ultrasound-guided nerve blocks are available. We sincerely hope that our practical and scientific experience, obtained over the past 15 years of clinical experience with ultrasound-guided regional anaesthesia, will further the worldwide enthusiasm in this field.

While modern learning tools, such as interactive DVDs, are available, there has yet to be published an anatomic textbook fulfilling the needs of anaesthetists interested in ultrasound anatomy. Cross-sectional anatomy is essential for ultrasound guidance in regional anaesthesia; irregular cross-sectional views are often required in order to perpendicularly visualize the targeted nerve. Furthermore, anatomic descriptions about the adjacent structures of nerves – with a clear focus on possible damages by the advancing needle – are needed. These descriptions should include ultrasound images with marked anatomic structures to enable better analysis of these images.

In contrast to the consensus over the need for new learning tools, certification of the use of ultrasonography in regional anaesthesia is a controversial topic. Some anaesthetists suggest a certification similar to the examinations in transesophageal echocardiography. However, while the introduction of mandatory exams might improve the quality of the techniques, it might hinder the uptake of ultrasound guidance. Moreover, potentially more dangerous, unguided-needle techniques are being performed without any additional qualifications required. A compromise might be a defined course of educational training for instructors, similar to that which currently exists for those working in advanced life support.

13.2 Technical developments

Ultrasonography has not been developed as a guidance technique for regional anaesthesia, the existing technique has simply been adapted by inventive anaesthesiologists to suit their needs. Nevertheless, ultrasound has a number of specific advantages for this purpose. One of the greatest benefits of ultrasound-guided regional anaesthesia is that fluids are extremely well visualized because of their hypoechoic appearance. Accordingly, the spread of local anaesthetic in human tissues is easy to detect. However, the technique also has specific problems, which may hinder its uptake in daily clinical practice. A major drawback of ultrasonography is that the ultrasound beam is extremely narrow, such that an inexperienced user will regularly lose sight of the needle while performing a nerve block. Even minimal changes in the position of the ultrasound probe can result in loss of needle visibility.

A possible solution to this would be the use of real-time 3D ultrasound probes ('4D'). Such probes are already available, and are currently used in echocardiography and obstetrics. Matrix-array ultrasound produces real-time 3D images by employing a square array of transducers to steer the ultrasound beam in 3D electronically with no moving parts. However, certain technical limitations mean that the currently available 3D probes are not suitable for ultrasound-guided nerve blockade. Firstly, the transducers in a regular 2D ultrasound probe have a linear array, and to reach a lateral resolution adequate for visualization of smaller structures, such as nerves, modern ultrasound probes carry 256 parallel transducers. In comparison, the transducers in 3D ultrasound probes are arranged in a 64×64 square and therefore have a lower lateral resolution. Secondly, the axial resolution of 3D probes presents another problem. These probes are used for relatively deep structures, such as a beating heart or a foetus. As such, their frequency is relatively low (approximately 4.5 MHz) and therefore they do not provide a suitable lateral resolution for most regional anaesthetic techniques.

Other medical applications, such as ultrasound-guided breast biopsy, are faced with the problem of needle guidance. The development of 3D ultrasound-guided breast biopsy systems is already at an advanced stage. High-resolution, real-time, 3D ultrasonography ('4D') will probably be available in the near future and will have a dramatic effect on the facilitation of ultrasound-guided regional anaesthesia. Furthermore, this new technology has the potential to further reduce the complication rate of regional anaesthesia, due to the improved visibility of the needle while advancing it through tissue close to the targeted neuronal structure.

Appendix 1

Zuers Ultrasound Experts Regional Anaesthesia Statement (ZUERS)

Participants

Chan Vincent, Department of Anaesthesia and Pain Management, University Health Network, Toronto Western Hospital, 399 Bathurst Street, MCL 2-405, Toronto, Ontario, Canada M5T 2S8, vchanvincent@cs.com

Greher Manfred, Department of Anaesthesiology, Perioperative Intensive Care and Pain Therapy, Herz-Jesu Hospital, Baumgasse 20A, A-1030 Vienna, Austria, m.greher@kh-herzjesu.at

Hollmann Markus, Academic Medical Center (AMC), University of Amsterdam, Department of Anaesthesia, Meibergdreef 9, NL-11005 DD Amsterdam, The Netherlands, m.w.hollmann@amc.uva.nl

Kapral Stephan, Medical University of Vienna, Department of Anaesthesia, General Intensive Care and Pain Control, Waehringer Guertel, 18–20, A-1090 Vienna, Austria, stephan.kapral@meduniwien.ac.at

Kettner Stephan, Medical University of Vienna, Department of Anaesthesia, General Intensive Care and Pain Control, Waehringer Guertel, 18–20, A-1090 Vienna, Austria, stephan.kettner@meduniwien.ac.at

Koscielniak-Nielsen Zbigniew, Department of Anaesthesia and Operative Services, 3033, HOC, Rigshospital, Blegdamsvej 9, 2100 Copenhagen, Denmark, zjkn@rh.dk

Lönnqvist Per-Arne, Paediatric Anaesthesia & Intensive Care, Astrid Lindgrens Children's Hospital, Karolinska University Hospital, SE-171 76 Stockholm, Sweden, per-arne.lonnqvist@ki.se

MacLeod David, Division of Orthopaedics, Plastics & Regional Anaesthesia, Department of Anaesthesiology, Duke University Medical Center, Durham NC 27710, USA, david.macleod@duke.edu

Marhofer Peter, Medical University of Vienna, Department of Anaesthesia, General Intensive Care and Pain Control, Waehringer Guertel, 18–20, A-1090 Vienna, Austria, peter.marhofer@meduniwien.ac.at

McCartney Colin, Department of Anaesthesia, Sunnybrook Health Sciences Centre, 2075 Bayview Avenue, Toronto, M4N3M5, Ontario, Canada, colin.mccartney@utoronto.ca

Nicholls Barry, Taunton & Somerset NHS Trust, Musgrove Park Hospital, Taunton, Somerset TA1 5DA, United Kingdom, barrynicholls@doctors.org.uk

Satoh Yutaka, Department of Anaesthesia, Goshogawara Municipal Hospital, 41 Nunoyamachi, Goshogawara City, 037-0053, Aomori, Japan, yuchan@sm.rim.or.jp

Weller Robert, Department of Anaesthesiology, Wake Forest University School of Medicine, Medical Center Blvd, Winston-Salem, NC 27157, USA, rweller@wfubmc.edu

Willschke Harald, Medical University of Vienna, Department of Anaesthesia, General Intensive Care and Pain Control, Waehringer Guertel, 18–20, A-1090 Vienna, Austria, harald.willschke@meduniwien.ac.at

Preamble

During the past ten years, ultrasound guidance for regional anaesthetic techniques has shown increasing popularity. Techniques for placing local anaesthetic adjacent to nerve structures have become more consistent with the use of ultrasound guidance, and the technology has been adopted by anaesthetists around the world. Despite this, there is little consistency and few recommendations as to what constitutes the best method to describe, perform, and teach many of these techniques. This could potentially hinder rather than promote the use of this valuable new technology, especially for new users.

A meeting of 14 experts from eight different countries and three continents, with a combined experience of many thousands of ultrasound-guided blocks, was convened in Zuers, Austria, in January 2007 to consider recommendations for promoting consistency in both the teaching and practice of ultrasound-guided regional anaesthesia. It was the aim of the group to promote the use of ultrasound by describing guidelines to facilitate performance of ultrasound-guided single-injection techniques in adults for regional anaesthesia and acute pain control. This encompassed recommendations for safe performance, grading of block performance difficulty, standardization of nomenclature for nerve visualization, and teaching recommendations. It was also recognized by the group that the evidence base for the use of these techniques is developing and that some of these recommendations may therefore be revised in the future, depending on further studies as they become available. These recommendations represent the opinions of a group of highly experienced practitioners and it is hoped that they may be of use to practitioners who are either starting to learn ultrasound-guided regional techniques or who wish to improve their existing skills.

The group did not consider the use of ultrasound for regional anaesthesia in children or for guidance of interventional pain relief procedures. These may be the subject of future recommendations.

Decision process

- Stage 1: Selection of expert panel based on one or more of the following criteria: Medline review, experience in education, significant clinical experience with ultrasound, special knowledge in regional anaesthesia.
- Stage 2: Identification of preliminary areas of importance in the field of ultrasonography in regional anaesthesia based on a survey 1 month prior to the expert meeting.
- Stage 3: Meeting in Zuers, Austria, January 7–12 2007.
- Stage 4: Post-meeting questionnaire of to help develop an ultrasound-guided block rating scale.
- Stage 5: Analysis of results and 3-month email-based discussion following the first draft of the expert statement.
- Stage 6: Final expert meeting statement.

Recommendations for appropriate, safe, and effective performance of ultrasound-guided techniques

- Start with basic block techniques.
- Use a machine and transducer capable of the highest-resolution imaging at the target depth.
- Optimize machine settings to visualize the nerve(s) whenever possible.
- Orient the transducer perpendicular (90°) to the anatomical course of the target structure(s) for optimal visualization.
- Maintain continuous awareness of the needle tip location.
- Choose a needle path that allows proximity of the needle tip to the nerve without needle–nerve contact.
- Immobile needle technique is suggested to allow careful maintenance of needle tip position during injection.
- Visualize the spread of local anaesthetic during injection. If no spread is visible, consider that intravascular injection may have occurred.
- Achieve circumferential spread of local anaesthetic where a discrete single nerve is visible. Limit further injection once circumneural spread is accomplished.
- Consider the use of a nerve stimulator to confirm nerve identity and to reduce the risk of intraneural injection if the target nerve structure is not clearly seen.

Definitions

Currently, various definitions of the 'position of the needle relative to the nerve' and the 'needle relative to the probe' are used. A uniform definition of the 'position of the needle relative to the nerve' and the 'needle relative to the probe' facilitates the understanding of future discussions and publications in the field of ultrasound-guided regional blocks.

Needle relative to the nerve

Figure A1 Short axis (SAX) position of the needle relative to the nerve

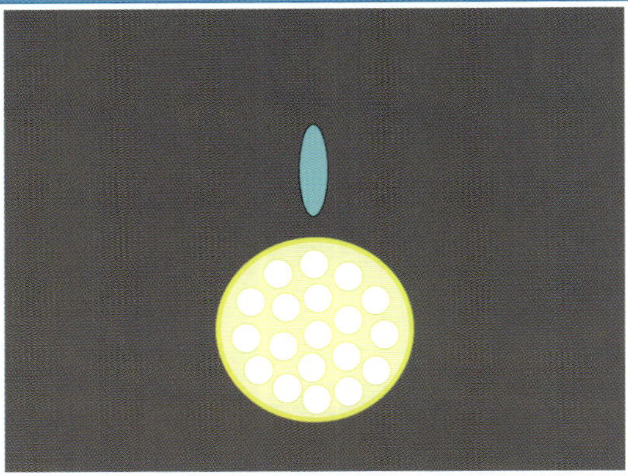

Figure A2 Long axis (LAX) position of the needle relative to the nerve

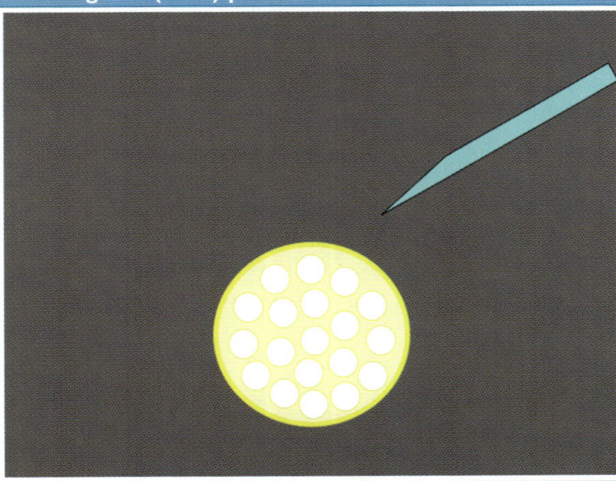

Needle relative to the probe

Figure A3 Out-of-plane position of the needle relative to the probe

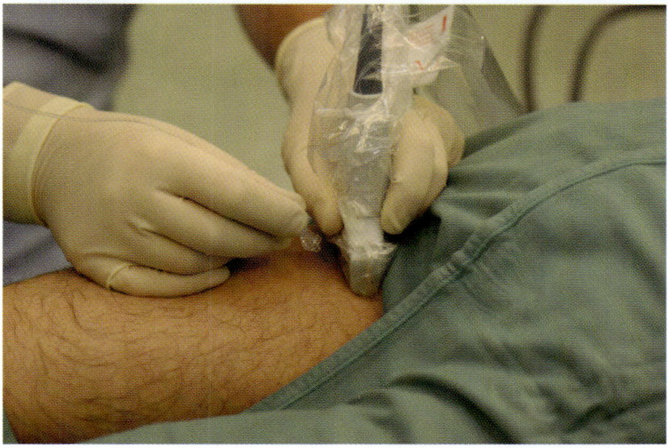

Figure A4 In-plane position of the needle relative to the probe

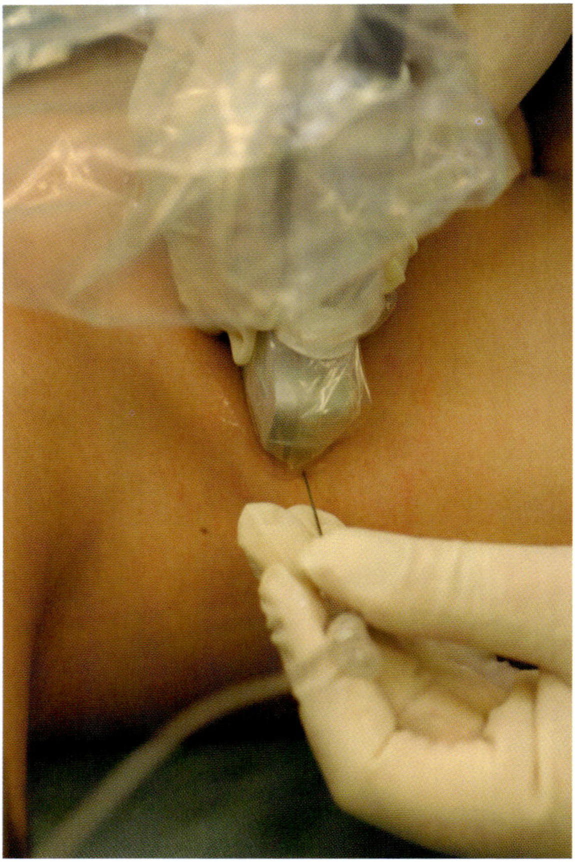

Training

- Basic knowledge of ultrasound physics and machine adjustment is required.
- Basic anatomy and sonoantomy of the relevant areas of interest is mandatory.
- An understanding of needle guidance techniques, as described in 'Definitions', is a prerequisite for safe and successful performance of regional blocks.
- Start with level 1 blocks.

Ultrasound-guided nerve block rating scale

This is a classification of ultrasound-guided peripheral nerve blocks, ranging from level 1 (basic) to level 3 (advanced), based upon the following four criteria:

- Ease of visualization of nerve structures (1: easy; 2: intermediate; 3: difficult)
- Ease of visualization of identifying feature(s) (1: easy; 2: intermediate; 3: difficult)
- Technical performance of block (1: easy; 2: intermediate; 3: difficult)
- Risk of complications from associated structures (1: low; 2: intermediate; 3: high).

Level I blocks (basic)

Superficial cervical, interscalene, axillary, terminal branches brachial plexus (ulnar/median/radial) – arm and forearm, femoral, saphenous, ankle blocks, ilioinguinal/iliohypogastric, rectus sheath.

Level II blocks (intermediate)

Supraclavicular, infraclavicular, obturator (anterior and posterior. branch), sciatic (subgluteal, midfemoral, and popliteal levels) posterior and lateral approaches, sciatic anterior approach, intercostal.

Level III blocks (advanced)

Deep cervical, lumbar plexus (posterior approach), thoracic paravertebral.

Table A1 Summary score based on the ultrasound-guided nerve block rating scale

Summary score	Level	Description
4–6	1	Basic
7–9	2	Intermediate
10–12	3	Advanced

Table A2 Definition of ultrasound probes

Definition of probe	Frequency
High frequency	> 10 MHz, linear
Medium frequency	6–10 MHz, linear
Low frequency	2–5 MHz, curved

Table A3 Particular peripheral regional anaesthetic techniques, probe recommendations and level of classification

Technique	Probe recommendation*	Summary score of 4 criterias (see above)**
Superficial cervical	High frequency, linear	6
Deep cervical	Medium frequency, linear	10
Interscalene	High frequency, linear	5
Supraclavicular	High frequency, linear	7
Infraclavicular	Medium frequency, linear	7
Axillary	High frequency, linear	6
Terminal branches brachial plexus (ulnar/median/radial)—arm and forearm	High frequency, linear	5
Femoral	High frequency, linear	5
Saphenous	High frequency, linear	6
Obturator (anterior and posterior branch)	High frequency, linear	7
Sciatic (subgluteal, midfemoral and popliteal levels), posterior and lateral approaches	Medium frequency, linear	7
Sciatic, anterior approach	Low frequency, curved	9
Ankle blocks	High frequency, linear	6
Lumbar plexus (posterior approach)	Low frequency, curved	11
Intercostal	High frequency, linear	8
Ilioinguinal/iliohypogastric	High frequency, linear	5
Rectus sheath	High frequency, linear	6
Thoracic paravertebral	Medium frequency, linear	10

* the recommendations are based on normal weight patients and may differ in obese patients.

** the summary score is the result of the mean evaluations of the 14 participants of the expert meeting.

Sterility

- Protect the probe and the cable with a cover to minimize patient–patient disease transmission.
- Aseptic needle insertion technique is recommended.

Machine requirements

- Adequate software for small-part ultrasonography.
- Data storage (still and video).
- Probes: see Table A2.
- High-frequency probes are appropriate for superficial blocks.

Needles

The following properties of needles are recommended:
- Short-bevel needles to facilitate needle tip visibility, especially for OOP insertion
- Needle length selection appropriate to the needle guidance technique (IP or OOP technique).
- Special echogenic needles demonstrate only a minor advantage, mainly for IP technique.

Needles whose aperture is set in some distance from the tip of the needle (e.g., Whitacre spinal or Sprotte needles) are not recommended because of the disproportion between the ultrasound-visible tip of the needle and the real outflow of local anaesthetic.

Conclusions and future directions

An expert statement in a relatively new field of interest can only serve as a current opinion. Experience and evidenced knowledge in ultrasound guidance is limited in comparison with more established techniques of nerve identification during regional blocks. Therefore, it is clear that the expert's opinions may be adapted in regular intervals. Nevertheless, safe and effective blocks should result from using these expert's opinions, in terms of recommendations, training, sterility, machine, and needle requirements. The expert statement should also work as a basis for future discussion and every user of these techniques is more than welcome to actively participate in developments in order to raise ultrasound guidance in regional anaesthesia to an adequate level of evidence that will ultimately ensure that the maximum number of patients profit from 'state of the art' techniques.

Appendix 2

Table A2 The Vienna score for ultrasound-guided nerve blocks

Score	Description
1	Internal structure of the nerve visualized
2	The nerve is visualized as a circular or oval-shaped bright halo (epineurium)
3	The nerve is visualized as reflections determined by the anatomy of the surrounded tissue
4	The anatomical position of the nerve shows no response to the ultrasound beam (isoechoic behaviour)

Index

M

N

O

P

R

S